TUBERCULOSIS OF THE LYMPHATIC SYSTEM

THE MACMILLAN COMPANY
NEW YORK · BOSTON · CHICAGO · DALLAS
ATLANTA · SAN FRANCISCO

MACMILLAN & CO., Limited
LONDON · BOMBAY · CALCUTTA
MELBOURNE

THE MACMILLAN CO. OF CANADA, Ltd.
TORONTO

TUBERCULOSIS

OF THE

LYMPHATIC SYSTEM

BY

WALTER BRADFORD METCALF, M.D.

ASSOCIATE IN CLINICAL MEDICINE, UNIVERSITY OF ILLINOIS, COLLEGE
OF MEDICINE. MEMBER, CONSULTING STAFF COOK COUNTY HOSPITAL,
CHICAGO MUNICIPAL TUBERCULOSIS SANITARIUM, LAKE GENEVA
SANITARIUM, VOLUNTEER MEDICAL SERVICE CORPS OF THE
UNITED STATES: FORMERLY, ATTENDING PHYSICIAN COOK
COUNTY HOSPITAL, DEPARTMENT OF TUBERCULOSIS

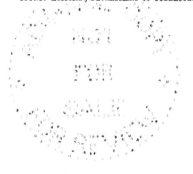

New York
THE MACMILLAN COMPANY
1919

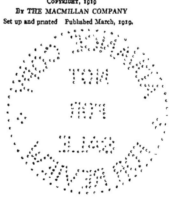

PREFACE

The following pages represent an attempt to emphasize the importance of glandular tuberculosis, especially as it occurs during childhood. Up to recent times there has been a tendency to consider this condition only as a local affair, but the modern view of considering the majority of cases of adult tuberculosis as autoinfections from old foci, contracted during childhood, places the question of glandular tuberculosis in another light. "Hilus tuberculosis" is an established entity. Tuberculous bronchial glands, the result of a childhood infection, undoubtedly are the most common source of adult pulmonary tuberculosis. The profession is just awakening to the fact that pulmonary tuberculosis of the adult can be prevented by proper prophylactic methods during childhood.

No condition so influences the development of the thorax as a tuberculous infection of the bronchial glands In fact, the entire development of the child is markedly influenced by such infection. There is increasing evidence that the so-called delicate and frail child is delicate and frail because of an existing tuberculous tracheo-bronchial adenopothy.

The surgeon is slowly giving up the field of tuberculous cervical adenitis. This condition should never be allowed to become a surgical question. Tuberculosis of the lymphatic system, especially during childhood, should be considered a serious affliction and be worthy of our best efforts, and if proper medical treatment is instituted during this primary stage of the infection nearly all cases will respond favorably—limit the course of the disease, and reduce its mortality.

A comparatively large space has been given to the subject of anatomy of the lymphatic system, the importance of which is seen when we begin to study the portals of entry of the infection, and the subsequent spreading of the disease.

In the treatment of tuberculosis the importance of fresh air, good food and hygienic surroundings is conceded by everyone. But the one agent, which in the author's opinion is the foremost weapon in our fight against tuberculosis, namely tuberculin, has been sadly neglected in our country.

In these pages a plea is made for the rational use of tuberculin as a diagnostic and therapeutic agent with special reference to its value in tuberculosis of the lymphatic system.

The author wishes to graciously express his appreciation for the able assistance rendered him by Assistant Surgeon Edwin Peterson, U. S. N. R. F. The many valuable references from French, German and Swedish medical literature were translated by him. He is also indebted to Dr. Roy M. Bowell for the compilation of parts of the subject-matter.

WALTER BRADFORD METCALF, M.D.

October, 1918

CONTENTS

TUBERCULOSIS OF THE LYMPHATIC SYSTEM

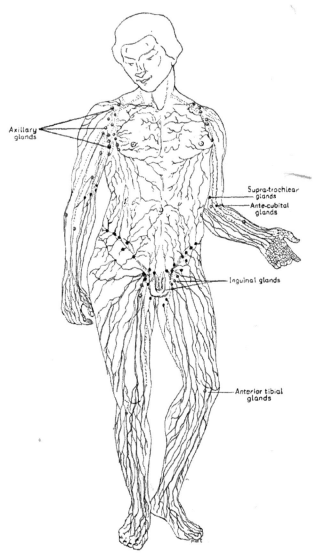

Axillary glands

Supra-trochlear glands

Ante-cubital glands

Inguinal glands

Anterior tibial glands

PLATE I.—SUPERFICIAL LYMPH-VESSELS. All superficial lymph-vessels are in black; the deep lymph-vessels throughout are colored red; afferent vessels are represented by continuous lines, and efferent vessels by dotted lines.

TUBERCULOSIS

OF THE LYMPHATIC SYSTEM

CHAPTER I

GENERAL ANATOMICAL CONSIDERATIONS

The Lymphatic System.—The development of the lymphatic
system has not been very well understood until recent years.
The close resemblance between the lymphatic vessels and the
veins has always been noted, but it was not until the last decade that the true relationship between the two systems was
established. Modern researches have proven conclusively that
the lymphatic system is a diverticulum from the veins and grows
into the organs by a process of budding.[1] The lymphatics hence
constitute a closed system which is lined throughout with endothelium. It resembles the bloodvascular system in many
points, but differs markedly in others. Like the latter, it is
made up of capillaries and larger vessels, but their contents
always flow in a centripetal direction, as is shown by the position of numerous valves and the gradual increase in size of the
vessels as they travel toward the neck, eventually emptying in
the larger veins of this region. (See Figure 1, Plate III.)
Another important difference is the presence of glands in the
course of the lymphatic vessels.

The Lymphatic Capillaries constitute blind sacs which dip
into the tissue spaces but are not continuous with them. They
anastomose freely with each other, the lymph travelling in the
direction of the least resistance. The lymphatic capillaries are,
as a rule, larger than the blood capillaries; their calibre varies
greatly within short distances. The capillaries are lined by a
single layer of nucleated endothelial cells with characteristic
crenated margins. By the union of the capillaries larger channels
are formed.

The Lymphatic Vessels Proper.—The close relationship between these vessels and the veins is clearly seen. In structure they resemble each other markedly. The endothelial linings are of the same character, but the muscular tissue in the wall of the lymphatic vessel is less in quantity. Numerous valves are present along the course of the vessels thus rendering backward flow of the lymph nearly impossible The vessel is somewhat dilated above each valve, giving it a beaded appearance. The lymphatic vessels collect the lymph from the different regions of the body, carry it through the lymph-glands, and after leaving the gland converge and form the terminal lymphatic trunks.

The Terminal Lymphatic Trunks.—The Jugular Trunk takes care of the lymph of the corresponding side of the head and neck and is formed by the union of the efferent vessels of the inferior deep cervical glands.

The Subclavian Trunk takes care of the lymph of the upper extremity of the corresponding side, draining the axillary glands.

The Broncho-mediastinal Trunk drains the lymph from the visceral lymphatic of the thorax and of the internal mammary chain.

The Right Lymphatic Duct.—The Termination of these trunks varies on the two sides. On the right side the three trunks may empty separately into the junction of the subclavian and internal jugular veins. The three vessels may converge and form the right lymphatic duct.

This Duct is more commonly formed by the union of the right subclavian and jugular, the broncho-mediastinal emptying separately. The right duct drains the right side of the head and neck, the right upper extremity, right side of thorax, right lung, right heart and convex surface of the liver.

On the left side the three trunks may empty into the thoracic duct, although this rarely occurs; the subclavian and broncho-mediastinal trunks usually converge or empty separately into the venous junction. The termination of each trunk is guarded by valves.

The Thoracic Duct conveys the mass of lymph from the greater part of the body into the blood; it is formed by the union

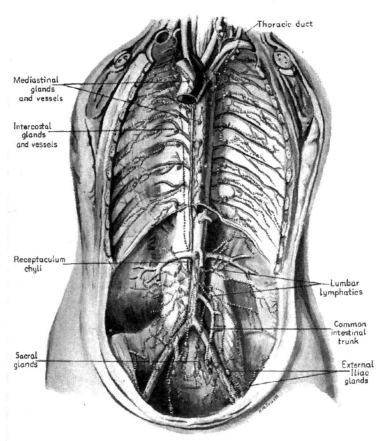

Thoracic duct

Mediastinal
glands
and vessels

Intercostal
glands
and vessels

Receptaculum
chyli

Lumbar
lymphatics

Common
intestinal
trunk

Sacral
glands

External
Iliac
glands

PLATE II.—A schematic presentation of the lymphatics of the thorax into the thoracic
duct, and the abdominal lymphatics into the receptaculum chyli.

PLATE III

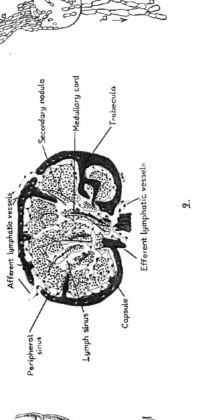

3.

A lymph-node showing its *afferent* and *efferent* vessels. a,a,a, the numerous *afferent* lymphatic vessels. b,b, the voluminous *efferent* vessels.

Secondary nodule

Medullary cord

Trabecula

Afferent lymphatic vessels

Efferent lymphatic vessels

Peripheral sinus

Lymph sinus

Capsule

2.

Diagrammatic section of a lymphatic node.

1.

Lymph-vessel laid open lengthwise, showing arrangement of valves preventing backward flow.

of the right and left lumbar trunks draining the retro-peritoneal organs, thus taking care of the lymph from the lower extremities, deep portions of the abdominal and pelvic walls. The intestinal trunk may enter at the same point draining the intra-peritoneal organs, thus pouring in the chyle from the small intestines.

The Triangular Dilatation, the receptaculum chyli, presents itself a little above the origin of the thoracic duct, thus being on a slightly higher level than the umbilicus, opposite to the first and second lumbar vertebræ.

The Thoracic Duct enters the thorax through the aortic opening of the diaphragm, lying to the right of the aorta. Opposite the fourth thoracic vertebra it inclines toward the left and ascends behind the arch of aorta and on the left side of the œsophagus to the upper orifice of the thorax; opposite the seventh cervical vertebra it turns outward between the vertebral and common carotid arteries and then downward over the subclavian artery to terminate in the left subclavian vein at the angle of junction with the left internal jugular vein.

The Duct averages about 45 c. m. in length and is provided with several valves, the most perfect being situated near its termination to prevent the regurgitation of the blood.

The Thoracic Duct drains the body below the diaphragm and the left side of the body above the diaphragm. It does not drain the convex surface of the liver.

The Lymphoid Tissue consists of reticular connective tissue and a special type of cells, the lymphoid cells which fill in the meshes of the reticulum. Lymphoid tissue may be diffuse or circumscribed. The diffuse type is found in the mucous membranes of the respiratory passages, throughout the intestinal tract, in the bone-marrow, etc. The circumscribed type may occur as solitary follicles in the intestinal mucosa or aggregated follicles (Peyers patches), especially in the lower end of the ileum.

The more complex structure of lymphoid tissue constitutes the lymphatic glands.

Lymphatic Glands are numerous and widely distributed bodies, which lie along the course of the lymphatic vessels. The number varies greatly in different individuals. They often occur in groups of from three to six, even ten to fifteen, forming chains which are placed in direct relation to the region which their afferent vessels drain.

The glands are usually rounded in form but may be elongated or cylindrical. In shape they somewhat resemble a bean, due to a concavity called the hilum, where the connective tissue of the capsule extends deeply into the substance of the node. This depression serves as point of entrance for the main arteries and nerves and of exit for the veins and efferent lymph-vessels. The afferent lymph-vessels enter on the convex side.

The glands are firm and elastic in consistency. They vary in size from the invisible to the size of an olive. Their color depends upon the location. They are, as a rule, whitish. The tracheo-bronchial glands are dark colored, due to the infiltration of small particles of coal, those of the liver yellow, etc. The glands are, as a rule, embedded in adipose connective tissue, in which they are easily movable.

On Miscroscopical Examination, the gland is shown to be surrounded by a distinct capsule, which externally is continuous with the cellulo-adipose tissue. The inner capsular layer sends prolongations into the gland substance from the hilum, forming the so-called trabeculæ. (See Figure 2, Plate III.)

The gland substance proper is separated from the capsule by the peripheral lymphatic sinus.

The outer portion of the gland, the cortex, is composed of regularly arranged lymph-nodules, trabeculæ and sinuses thus distinguishing it from the medulla. The center of each nodule is the seat of active proliferation of the lymphoid cells, thus forming the Germinal Center.

The central portion of the gland, the medulla, is made up of strands of lymphoid tissue, the lymph-cords, which extend from the nodules of the cortex forming an irregular mass of tissue. Hence the difference between the cortex and medulla is only one of degree.

The reticular network forms part of the lymphatic tissue proper and is continuous with the connective tissue of the trabeculæ and capsule.   The reticulum serves as a meshwork for the lymphoid cells which nearly obscure it in the nodules.

The Afferent Lymphatics, entering the gland on its convex surface, form a plexus of capillaries, which by their anastomoses produce the peripheral sinus.   From this sinus internodular branches run towards the medulla, anastomosing freely with each other throughout the glandular substance.   Thus the lymphoid tissue is bathed on nearly every side with lymph.   In the hilum of the gland the sinuses collect into the terminal sinus, which communicates with the efferent lymphatics, leaving at the hilum.   (See Figure 3, Plate III)

The Blood Supply.—The gland receives blood supply from two sources, through the hilum and through the convex surface of the capsule.   The arteries entering through the hilum are the larger and ramify along the trabeculæ, giving off numerous branches, finally being resolved into a very rich capillary network, which extends into the cortical lymph-nodules and the medullary lymph-cords.

The vessels entering through the convex surface of the gland supply the capsule and trabeculæ anastomosing in some cases with the other group.

The nerve supply consists of both non-medullated and medullated fibers; their exact significance is uncertain—some of them are without question vasomotor in character.

CHAPTER II

ANATOMICAL RÉSUMÉ OF THE MOST IMPORTANT GLANDULAR CHAINS AND AREAS OF LYMPHATIC DRAINAGE OF HEAD AND NECK

The profound studies of the lymphatic system, made many years ago by SAPPEY, stand the test of modern investigations. DELAMERE, POIRIER and CUNEO,[2] basing their work upon that of SAPPEY, have added many facts to our knowledge of the lymphatic apparatus.

In more recent years BEITZKE, MOST,[3] P. BARTELS,[4] W. S. MILLER,[8, 9] G. SCHWEITZER and others, have made extensive researches with respect to the lymph-passages. The following facts are mainly drawn from the works of these modern investigators.

LYMPHATIC GLANDS OF HEAD AND NECK

The Occipital Glands are two to three in number on each side of the median line, between the anterior border of the Trapezius and insertion of the Complexus. They drain the occipital region of the scalp and send their efferent vessels down to the deep cervical glands.

The Auricular Glands may be divided into the three following groups:

The Pre-auricular Glands are, as a rule, one to two in number and are located just in front of the tragus. They drain the anterior and upper part of the external ear and the anterior temporal region of the scalp; their efferent vessels go to the parotid glands.

The Infra-auricular Glands are located just beneath the ear and are one to two in number; they drain the inferior part of the external ear and send their efferent vessels to the parotid glands.

The Retro-auricular Glands, also called the Mastoid Glands, are situated just beneath the border of the Retrahens aurem

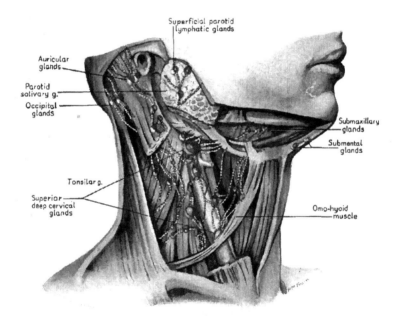

Superficial parotid
lymphatic glands

Auricular
glands

Parotid
salivary g.

Occipital
glands

Submaxillary
glands

Submental
glands

Tonsilar g.

Superior
deep cervical
glands

Omo-hyoid
muscle

PLATE IV.—A schematic drawing showing the drainage from the superficial lymphatics of
the head to the deep lymphatics in the neck, in accordance with descriptions.

muscle. They drain the posterior surface of the external ear and the adjacent region of the scalp and send their efferent vessels down to the deep cervical glands. .

The Parotid Lymph-glands may be divided into two groups with reference to their relation to the parotid salivary gland.

The Superficial Parotid Glands are situated just beneath the fascia, partially embedded in the superficial layers of the salivary gland; their afferent vessels arise from the anterior surface of the external ear, root of the nose, forehead, eyelids, upper part of the cheek, anterior temporal portion of the scalp and from some of the auricular glands. The efferent vessels pass mainly to the deep and superficial cervical glands.

The Deep Parotid Glands are situated in the substance of the salivary gland and are usually two to four in number. They drain the ocular conjunctiva, deep portion of the forehead, root of the nose and temporal region of the scalp and the substance of the parotid salivary gland. The efferent vessels pass into the superficial and deep cervical glands

The Superficial Cervical Lymph-glands are three to four in number and lie beneath the superficial cervical fascia on the Sterno-cleido-mastoid muscle, near the angle of the jaw in the region of the external jugular vein. They drain the parotid region of the face and the external ear. They also receive the lymph from the submaxillary, parotid and auricular glands; the efferent vessels go to the deep cervical glands.

The Submaxillary Lymph-glands are located in the sub-maxillary triangle along the anterior border of the mandible, resting on the submaxillary salivary gland. Their number and position are, according to MOST, very constant. They consist of three glands or gland groups which BARTELS has named the anterior, middle and posterior.

The Anterior Gland lies in the anterior angle of the submaxillary triangle on the Mylohyoid muscle near the anterior belly of the Digastric muscle on the submental vein.

The Mesial Gland is, as a rule, the largest and is located along the border of the lower jaw just mesially to the external maxillary artery.

The **Posterior Gland** lies, as a rule, laterally to the anterior facial vein.

The **Submaxillary Lymph-glands** take care of the lymph from the largest part of the face, especially the lips, external nose, cheeks, anterior part of the lids, floor of the mouth, teeth and gums, mucous membranes of the cheeks and anterior part of the mucous membrane of the nose. The efferent vessels pass into the superficial and deep cervical glands.

The **Submental Lymph-glands** are one to four in number and are located in the triangle bounded by the anterior bellies of the Digastric muscles and the Hyoid bone. They drain the integument of the chin, central portion of the skin of the lower lip, the mucous membrane of the corresponding portion of the alveolar border of the mandible, the floor of the mouth and the tip of the tongue. The efferent vessels pass into the submaxillary lymph-glands.

The **Retro-pharyngeal Lymph-glands** are usually two in number and located behind the pharynx, at the junction of its posterior and lateral surface, on a level with the Atlas. The afferent vessels come from the muscles and fascia in front of the vertebræ, nasal fossæ and accessory cavities, nasopharynx, eustachian tube and possibly from the cavity of the tympanum. The efferent vessels pass into the deep cervical glands.

The **Deep Cervical Glands** are numerous, fifteen to thirty in number, lying along the carotid artery and internal jugular vein. The chain extends from the apex of the mastoid process of the temporal bone to the junction of the internal jugular and subclavian veins; they may be divided into the following groups and subgroups:

The **Superior Deep Cervical Glands** are located on the lateral side of the neck, especially in the superior carotid triangle and the upper part of the occipital triangle; this part of the chain hence extends from the tip of the mastoid process to the region, where the common carotid artery is crossed by the Omohyoid muscle.

The **Mesial group** is located in the superior carotid triangle in immediate vicinity of the large vessels.

The Lateral group is located in the upper angle of the occipital triangle.

The Superior Deep Cervical Glands take care of the lymph from the head and all the parts of the upper neck region. The efferent vessels pass into the inferior deep cervical glands.

The Inferior Deep Cervical Glands are also called the Supra-clavicular Glands and lie below the Omohyoid muscle in the subclavian triangle.

The Mesial Group comprises a few glands which lie behind the internal jugular vein. The efferent vessels from this group unite with some from the superior mesial group; the collecting vessels finally unite and form the jugular trunk or empty directly into the thoracic duct or right lymphatic duct respectively. The lateral group is located in the subclavian triangle proper. These glands are connected with the superior lateral group and also with the axillary lymph-glands. The efferent vessels help to form the jugular trunk.

The Inferior Deep Cervical Glands take care of the lymph from the lower neck region, especially the thyroid gland and in-directly from the part drained by the superior deep cervical glands, also from the pretracheal glands. The efferent vessels form the jugular trunk from where the lymph passes to the tho-racic duct or right lymphatic duct respectively.

The Prelaryngeal Glands usually lie on the middle crico-thyroid ligament between the two Crico-thyroid muscles. They drain the anterior part of the larynx, from the free border of the vocal cords, downwards to the beginning of the trachea, also part of the thyroid gland; the efferent vessels pass into the deep cervical and pretracheal glands.

The Pretracheal Glands are located below the isthmus of the thyroid in front of the trachea; they are of small size and usually one to three in number; the afferent vessels come from the thyroid and prelaryngeal glands; the efferent vessels empty into the supraclavicular glands.

AREAS OF LYMPHATIC DRAINAGE OF HEAD AND NECK

The Skin.—From the forehead, nose, lips and chin region, the lymph travels to the submental and submaxillary lymph-glands; the further back we come on the lateral surface of the face, the more regularly are the parotid glands interposed and even the superficial cervical glands; the deep cervical lymph-glands constitute the second station for this area.

The Eye.—The External Eye: The lymph-vessels of the eye-lids and the conjunctiva form two parts:

The mesial vessels correspond to the angular artery and collect the lymph from the internal half of the eyelids and conjunctiva and pass, as a rule, to the submaxillary lymph-glands.

The lateral vessels correspond to the transverse facial artery. They arise from the greatest part of the upper eyelid, lateral half of the lower and corresponding part of the conjunctiva and run to the parotid lymph-glands.

The Internal Eye: No true lymphatic vessels have been demonstrated in the sclera, lens or vitreous humor.

The Ear.—The External Ear is drained by the auricular and deep cervical glands.

The Middle Ear and Auditory Canal: The auricular glands drain the lateral portion; the retro-pharyngeal and deep cervical the mesial portion.

The Internal Ear: Nothing is known of its lymphatics.

The Nasal Cavity.—The lymph of the nares travels in two directions: from the most anterior part it goes to the submaxillary glands, but the main stream of lymph from the posterior portion travels along the lateral wall of the pharynx to the lateral retro-pharyngeal and the deep cervical glands.

Little is known of the lymphatics of the accessory sinuses of the nose. The lymph from the frontal sinus is taken care of by the lateral retro-pharyngeal and the deep cervical glands; the lymphatics of the superior maxillary sinus travel to the submaxillary glands.

The Gums.—The lymph-vessels of the gums have been studied

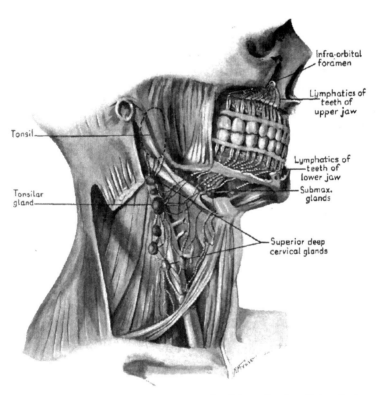

Infra-orbital
foramen

Lymphatics of
teeth of
upper jaw

Tonsil

Lymphatics of
teeth of
lower jaw

Submax.
glands

Tonsilar
gland

Superior deep
cervical glands

PLATE V.—A schematic presentation of the lymphatics of the teeth and tonsils into the deep
tonsillar gland.

by G. SCHWEITZER, whose results P. BARTELS summarizes as follows:

"The gums are traversed by an extremely fine and delicate network of lymphatic capillaries; from these, two groups of vessels arise.

"The outer group forms a plexus, which encircles the alveolar processes of the jaws along the lower and upper folds of the mucous membrane and forms mesial anastomoses. The regional lymph-glands are the submaxillary, submental and deep cervical glands.

"The inner vessels of the gums of the upper jaw travel through the mucous membrane of the hard palate, or over the soft palate and pharyngeal wall downwards toward the deep cervical glands. In the lower jaw the vessels from the incisor region travel to the anterior submaxillary glands and the balance to the deep cervical glands."

The Teeth.—The existence of lymphatics in the tooth-pulp has long been denied until G. SCHWEITZER succeeded in demonstrating them. He says, "The presence of lymphatics in the pulp of the fully developed and embryonal teeth has been demonstrated, but their number and course are not yet completely established."

The collecting vessels from the teeth of the upper jaw most probably unite and pass through the infra-orbital foramen and travel to the submaxillary glands.

The regional lymph-glands of the teeth of the lower jaw have not been demonstrated absolutely, but from analogy, with the lymphatics of the gums, it may be concluded that they are the submaxillary and deep cervical glands. (See Schweitzer's Table, p. 12.)

The Oral Cavity.—The lymph-vessels of the mouth pass mainly to the submaxillary and superficial cervical glands. From the main part of the tongue, and posterior part of the oral cavity, the lymph goes to the mesial group of the superior deep cervical glands.

The Throat.—The lymphatics of the upper and posterior region of the throat travel to the retro-pharyngeal glands, whence

SCHWEITZER'S TABLE

From region of	The upper jaw to the submaxillary glands			The lower jaw to the submaxillary glands		
	Anter. Gl.	Mesial Gl.	Post. Gl.	Anter. Gl.	Mesial Gl.	Post. Gl.
Incisors	Occasionally one vessel	About $5/6$	About $1/6$	About $1/3$	About $2/3$	Occasionally one vessel
Premolars	o	about $2/3$	about $1/3$	seldom one vessel	nearly all	o
Molars	o	nearly $1/2$	somewhat more than $1/2$	occasionally one vessel	nearly all	occasionally one vessel

they go to the deep cervical glands. The lymph from the lateral walls of the pharynx, especially from the tonsillar region, is taken care of by the mesial group of the deep cervical glands.

Lymph-vessels from the anterior and lower part of the throat penetrate the thyreo-hyoid membrane and join the vessels from the region of epiglottis and larynx and arrive at the mesial group of the deep cervical glands.

The Larynx.—The lymph-vessels from the upper portion of the larynx travel the same route as the vessels from the anterior and lower part of the pharynx, penetrate the thyreo-hyoid membrane and go to the mesial group of the deep cervical glands.

The lymph from the region of the anterior subglottal space is taken care of by delicate vessels which penetrate the crico-thyreo-hyoid membrane and go to the laryngeal glands, while the lymphatics of the mucous membrane of the posterior wall of the larynx go to the pretracheal glands.

TONSILLAR RING OF WALDEYER

The ensemble of lymphoid tissue, the palatine, lingual and pharyngeal tonsils, situated at the entrance of the respiratory and digestive passages, form an almost complete ring commonly known as "Waldeyer's ring."

The Palatine Tonsil or Faucial Tonsil.—The Palatine Tonsil consists of a rounded mass of lymphoid tissue on each side of the fauces. The tonsil varies markedly in size, but in the young adult averages about twenty m. m. in height, fifteen m. m. in width and twelve m. m. in thickness. The lateral surface is covered by the capsule which is continuous with the pharyngeal aponeurosis. The pharyngeal surface is covered with the mucous membrane of the pharynx and presents the openings of various crypts, twelve to fifteen in number, lined with stratified epithelium.

The Blood Supply.—The tonsils are very rich in blood supply. The most important arteries are the ascending palatine and tonsillar branches of the facial artery, dorsalis linguæ of the lingual, ascending pharyngeal of the external carotid and the descending palatine branch of the internal maxillary artery.

The Lymphatics of the Tonsils are not well understood. HENKLE [5] in a recent rather remarkable series of experiments tried to prove that the tonsils were concerned in draining the mucous membrane of the nose and gums, thus substantiating the findings of V. LENART, FRANKEL and WRIGHT. But KARL AMERSBACH [6] has still more recently reported the results of his own experiments carried out in nearly the same manner as HENKLE'S, except as G. B. WOOD [7] remarks, that he was more careful in the method of injection. In his experiments on human beings he injected carbon pigments into the mucosa of the nose and mouth and was in no instance able to recover any part of them in the tonsils. In his experiments on dogs he showed that these particles travelled down to the submaxillary glands, hence along a route anatomically demonstrated by our foremost anatomists.

G. B. WOOD'S contention is thus upheld that as far as we know there are no afferent lymph-vessels running to the parenchyma of the tonsils; neither have any perilymphatic spaces been demonstrated. The efferent lymph-vessels empty into the superior deep cervical glands, especially the so-called tonsillar gland, lying under the anterior border of the Sterno-cleido-mastoid muscle, just behind the angle of the mandible.

The Functions of the Tonsils, as that of the Waldeyer's Ring in general is, from their important anatomical position, to be considered as one of direct defense against microbic invasion. Absorption through the intact tonsillar epithelium is a disputed question.

According to some investigations the tonsils per se actually antagonize the entrance to their interior of infectious germs. But if they are once absorbed the anatomical structure of the gland will delay their passage, thus giving the ever present leucocytes a chance to exercise their phagocytic power. Another protective function of the tonsil is possibly shown by the so-called Stöhr's phenomena; the tonsils are traversed by an enormous number of leucocytes which exercise a kind of migration toward the oral cavity. Some investigators believe that the tonsils have an internal secretion but exact proof of its existence is, as yet, wanting.

The Lingual Tonsils are small lymphatic organs situated on either side of the central line at the base of the tongue; each tonsil has usually one crypt, lined with a continuation of the surface stratified squamous epithelium.

The Pharyngeal Tonsils, or Tonsils of Luschka, consist of a mass of lymphoid tissue lying in the vault of the naso-pharynx. They are covered by columnar ciliated epithelium. Hypertrophy of these tonsils constitutes what is known as adenoids.

Visceral Lymphatic Glands of the Thorax

The painstaking research on the lymphoid tissue in the lung, as done by W. S. MILLER,[8] is of interest in that it shows the minute development of the lymphatic system in the lung proper and the distribution of lymphoid tissue in its relation to the bronchi, blood and lymph-vessels and the pleura. The lymphoid tissue in the lung may be in the form of lymph-nodes, lymph-follicles or small masses of lymphoid tissue. Lymph-nodes in the normal lung are found associated with the larger divisions of the bronchi. They are situated at the place where branching takes place. In the normal lung lymph-nodes are not present in the pleura.[8]

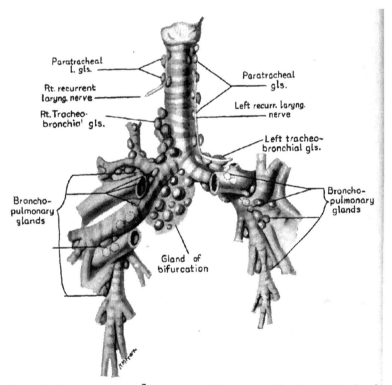

PLATE VI.—Glands in relation to the trachea and the large bronchi. (After Lukiennikow.)

The smaller masses of lymphoid tissue may, like the lymph-nodes, act as filters interpolated in the lymph circulation. They also serve as centres to which the phagocytes carry their collected material. According to MILLER [9] the flow in the lymphatics of the bronchi, of the arteries, of the main venous trunks and the greater part of the pleura is toward the hilum of the lung. In the lymphatics about the veins, the flow, in those vessels which are situated just beneath the pleura and communicate with the pleural network of lymphatics, may be towards the pleura.

The Visceral Lymph-glands of the Thorax form two main groups—the mediastinal and bronchial, which are divided into the following sub-groups.

The Anterior Mediastinal Glands are located in the anterior mediastinum in front of the aorta and left innominate vein. They are six to seven in number and drain the heart, pericardium, thymus gland, anterior mediastinum and a great part of the liver. The efferent vessels pass into the right and left broncho-mediastinal trunks respectively.

The Posterior Mediastinal Glands lie behind the pericardium along the thoracic aorta; they drain the posterior portion of the diaphragm and pericardium and send their efferent vessels to the right and left lymphatic ducts.

The Bronchial Glands are extremely numerous and are, according to their location, divided into the following sub-groups:

The Tracheo-bronchial Lymph-glands are situated in the lateral angles, between the trachea and the bronchus on each side. Their afferent vessels come from the other group of bronchial glands and adjacent parts of the trachea and bronchi. The efferent vessels pass to the broncho-mediastinal trunk; occasionally one vessel passes to the lateral group of the supraclavicular glands.

Lymph-glands of the Bifurcation are located in the angle between the two main bronchi. They are nine to twelve in number and drain the adjacent parts; they also receive the efferent vessels of the broncho-pulmonary glands; their efferent vessels pass to the tracheo-bronchial glands.

The Broncho-pulmonary Glands are embedded in the hilus of the lung and drain the lung substance directly or through the pulmonary glands; their efferent vessels may go directly to the tracheo-bronchial glands, or via those of the bifurcation.

The Pulmonary Lymph-glands are situated in the lung substance which they drain; the efferent vessels pass into the broncho-pulmonary glands.

Lymphatic Glands of the Abdomen

The Mesenteric Glands are the most important. They are located between the layers of the mesentery and vary in number from 100 to 250. They form three main groups, the outer, middle and inner.

The outer group lies close to the wall of the small intestines and contains the smallest glands.

The middle group consists of somewhat larger glands and corresponds in position to the narrowing of the mesentery toward its root.

The inner group lies on the root of the mesentery and contains the largest glands.

The Mesenteric Glands take care of the lymph from the small intestine except the duodenum and receive the efferent vessels from the mesocolic and ileo-cæcal glands. The efferent channels pass to the intestinal trunk.

The Mesocolic Glands are found between the layers of the mesentery of the large intestine; they are from 20 to 30 in number and receive their afferent vessels from the large intestine, sending their efferent ones to the mesenteric lymph-glands.

The Cæcal Lymph-glands may be divided into the following groups:

The Pre-cæcal, on the anterior surface of the cæcum, the Retro-cæcal, on the posterior surface of the cæcum, and the Ileo-cæcal surrounding the termination of the ileo-cæcal artery.

The Lymph from the cæcum is sent to the pre-cæcal and retro-cæcal glands, from where it passes to the ileo-cæcal and mesenteric glands.

The **Appendicular Lymph-glands** are very inconsistent as to location and number; they surround the appendicular artery and drain the appendix sending their efferent vessels to the ileo-cæcal glands.

The **Gastric Glands.**—The Superior Gastric Glands lie between the folds of the lesser omentum along the lesser curvature of the stomach, following the course of the right and left gastric arteries.

The inferior Gastric Glands are located in the folds of the gastro-colic ligaments along the greater curvature following the course of the right and left gastro-epiploic arteries.

The glands take care of the lymph from the walls of the stomach and send their efferent vessels to the pancreatico-splenic glands from where it passes to the cœliac glands.

The **Hepatic Glands** lie in the hepato-duodenal ligament along the course of the hepatic artery and receive their afferent vessels from the liver and gall bladder, pylorus, duodenum and head of the pancreas. The efferent vessels pass to the cœliac glands.

The **Pancreatico-splenic Glands** are located behind the pancreas in the hilum of the spleen between the folds of the gastro-splenic ligament along the splenic artery. They receive the lymph from the pancreas, duodenum, liver, stomach and spleen and send their efferent vessels into the cœliac glands.

The **Cœliac Lymph-glands** form the upper intestinal glands and lie behind the pancreas, duodenum and pylorus, in front of the abdominal aorta, between and behind the layers of the transverse mesocolon and lesser omentum. They receive the lymph from the digestive organs, lying above the transverse mesocolon, having previously passed through intermediate lymph-glands. The efferent vessels help to form the intestinal lymphatic trunk.

The **Lumbar Lymph-glands** are situated on the posterior wall of the abdomen behind the parietal peritoneum, in front of the Psoas major and Quadratus lumborum muscles and surround the abdominal aorta, especially on its posterior surface. These glands receive the efferent vessels of the iliac, hypo-gastric, sacral and mesocolic glands, and afferent vessels from the kidneys, adrenals, testicles, fundus of uterus, tubes and ovaries, the deep back muscles and from the under surface of the vertebral part of the diaphragm. Their efferent vessels go to form the lateral tributaries of the thoracic duct—namely, the right and left lumbar trunks.

LYMPHATIC GLANDS OF THE PELVIS

The Ano-Rectal Glands are located in the lower part of the true pelvis on the lateral sides of the rectum; their efferent vessels convey the lymph from the mucous membrane and muscular coat of the rectum and from the mucous membrane of the upper part of the anal canal; the efferent vessels pass into the superior hemorrhoidal glands.

The Para-uterine Glands are embedded in the folds of the broad ligament close to the neck of the uterus, which organ they also drain; the efferent vessels pass into the hypo-gastric lymph-glands.

The Vesicular Glands are located on the anterior and lateral walls of the bladder, the walls of which organ they also drain, sending their efferent vessels into the external iliac glands.

The Hemorrhoidal Glands lie in the meso-rectum following the course of the superior hemorrhoidal artery; these glands drain the pelvic part of the rectum and receive the efferent vessels of the ano-rectal glands, sending their own efferents to the inferior mesenteric glands.

The Sacral Glands are located on the anterior surface of the sacrum. They take care of the lymph from the adjacent wall of the pelvis, the afferent vessels anastomosing with those of the rectum and prostate gland; the efferent vessels pass to the hypogastric and lumbar glands.

The Hypogastric Glands lie on the lateral walls of the pelvis, following the course of the hypogastric vessels; the afferent vessels receive lymph from the gluteal region, hip joint, internal surface of the thigh, perineum, urogenital tract, upper third of the vagina, uterus, prostate gland, seminal vesicles and rarely from the penis. The efferent vessels are sent to the common iliac and lumbar glands.

The **Iliac Glands** follow the course of the external and common iliac vessels from the femoral ring to the fifth lumbar vertebra. They receive the efferent vessels of the inguinal glands, especially Rosenmuller's gland, the inferior epigastric and the hypogastric glands; the iliac glands also drain the penis, clitoris, vagina, bladder and the abdominal wall below the umbilicus; the efferent vessels go into the lumbar glands.

Lymph-glands of the Upper Extremities

The **Antibrachial Glands** lie along the course of the radial and ulnar arteries.

The **Superficial Cubital** or the **Supra-trochlear Glands** are located just above the medial epicondyle to the mesial side of the basilic vein where it pierces the deep fascia.

The **Deep Cubital Glands** lie deep in the cubital region near the large vessels.

The **Axillary Glands** drain the upper part of the thoracic wall and the upper extremities; they vary markedly in number from eight or ten, to fifty or more. P. BARTELS divides them into the following groups:

The **Pectoral Glands** are located along the lower border of the Pectoralis major muscle and drain the mammary gland and front and side of thorax; they send their efferent vessels into the intermediate and infra-clavicular groups.

The **Subscapular Glands** follow closely the subscapular vessels and receive their afferent vessels from the dorsal surface of the thorax. The efferent vessels pass to the brachial group.

The **Brachial Glands** lie the deepest of the axillary glands behind the axillary vessels and receive the lymph from the superficial and deep lymphatics of the arm; they send their efferent vessels to the intermediate and infra-clavicular groups.

The **Subpectoral Glands** are located beneath the Pectoralis minor muscle to the mesial side of the axillary vessels, draining the region supplied by the acromio-thoracic artery.

The **Intermediate or Central Glands** are situated deep in the axilla along the axillary artery below the origin of the long thoracic artery; they receive the efferent vessels of the other groups, sending their own to the infra-clavicular group.

The Infra-clavicular Glands lie between the upper border of the Pectoralis minor muscle and the clavicle to the mesial side of the subclavian vein. The efferent vessels unite to form the subclavian trunk: anastomosis does sometimes exist with the supra-clavicular glands.

Lymphatic Glands of the Lower Extremities

The Anterior Tibial, The Popliteal and the Posterior Tibial Glands take care of the lymph of the lower extremity sending it through the inguinal glands.

The Inguinal Glands are divided into the superficial and deep groups: the former is divided in two sub-groups, the superficial inguinal and superficial sub-inguinal.

The Superficial Inguinal Glands are located above a line drawn through the point where the saphenous vein pierces the fascia of the fossa ovalis. They lie just below Poupart's ligament.

The Superficial Sub-inguinal Glands are located just below the above mentioned line.

The Superficial Group drain the skin of the lower extremity, the gluteal region, perineum, abdominal wall, scrotum, anus, prepuce of clitoris, and sometimes glans penis and clitoris. The efferent vessels pass into the external iliac glands.

The Deep Inguinal Glands lie beneath the fascia lata. They are small in size and few in number. The gland of Rosenmuller is the largest and is located in the femoral ring. These glands receive some of the efferent vessels of the superficial groups and send their own channels to the iliac glands.

CHAPTER III

PHYSIOLOGICAL CONSIDERATIONS

Composition of the Lymph.—RUDBECK, one of the discoverers of the lymphatic system (1653) said that the lymph is a water-clear liquid of salty taste which coagulates spontaneously. TIGERSTEDT remarks that our present knowledge is not much more complete.

The chemical composition of lymph corresponds to that of the blood plasma with slight variations in the albumen contents. TIGERSTEDT gives the following percentage composition of human lymph: [10]

Water........93–96%

Solids........ 4– 7%
$\begin{cases} \text{Fibrin}\dots\dots\dots\dots\dots\dots 0.04\text{–}0.05\% \\ \text{Albumen}\dots\dots\dots\dots\dots 3.5\text{ –}4.3\ \% \\ \text{Inorganic salts (ashes)}\dots\dots 0.7\text{ –}0.8\ \% \\ \text{Fat}\dots\dots\dots\dots\dots\dots 0.4\text{ –}0.9\ \% \\ \text{Cholesterin and Lecithin} \end{cases}$

In examining the lymph from a dog, HAMMERSTEN found only traces of oxygen but about 42 vol.% of carbonic acid; hence a greater quantity than in the arterial blood but less than in the venous.

Microscopical Examination of the Lymph.—Microscopical examination of the lymph reveals the presence of white blood-cells in varying numbers and a few red blood-cells.

During recent years many investigations have been made as to the physiological action of the lymph itself. ASHER and BARBERA reinjected neck lymph secured by passive massage of the neck, into the central end of the internal carotid artery and found some changes in the blood pressure. According to the same authors, the substance in the lymph producing these effects on the vasomotor centre, is produced in the tissue and rendered innocuous or ineffective in the lymph-glands; massage of the head and neck prevented this in the experiments. CARLSON, GREER and BECHT [11] proved that the lymph itself has a lymphagogue action, probably due to the presence of a hormone produced in the normal activity of the tissues.

Circulation of the Lymph.—The movement of the lymph is always a centripetal one, from the radicals of the lymphatic system toward the larger vessels. Many factors are concerned in the circulation of the lymph. The tissue tension without question plays an important rôle. When the tissue-liquid is increased, the tissue tension is consequently raised and thus the lymph-stream accentuated. Muscular contraction produces the same result, increasing the tissue-tension. The upward movement of the lymph in the thoracic duct is mainly caused by the inspiratory act producing a negative pressure in the thoracic cavity. The presence of valves removes the possibility of backward flow.

Formation of the Lymph.—The formation of lymph is as yet a disputed question. The old theory defended by LUDWIG and his pupils, taught that the lymph was derived from the blood-plasma by a simple process of filtration, depending upon the greater pressure in the blood-channels. But recent investigations seem to disprove this conception.

The difference in pressure and osmotic tension between the arterial capillaries and the surrounding tissue and lymphatic radicals is undoubtedly a partial factor in formation of the lymph, but CARLSON, GREER and LUCKHARD [12] showed that the chloride content in the lymph was larger than in the blood, thus rendering the filtration and transudation theories of lymph-formation untenable.

HEIDENHAIM proved that the injection of certain substances, lymphagogues, into the blood-stream resulted in increased lymph-formation without increasing the blood pressure. He proposed the theory that the cells of the capillary walls have a secretory function, thus being partially responsible for the lymph-formation.

ASHER has still more recently emphasized the relation between lymph-formation and the activity of the tissues; he considers the lymph a product, a secretion of the functionating tissue cells.

CARLSON, GREER and BECHT propose the theory that one of the normal mechanisms of lymph-formation is a hormone, produced in the normal activity of the tissues and acting by augmenting the normal secretory activity of the capillary endothelium.

According to some authors the phenomena observed in the lymph-formation can be explained by physical-chemical laws. STARLING [13] believes that the lymphagogue action of certain substances depends upon an injurious effect upon the capillary endothelium, thus rendering it more permeable.

The Lymphatic Vessels and their Function.—The lymph-vascular system may be regarded as a drainage apparatus, which takes care of the excessive liquid present in the body tissues. In many tissues the lymph-vessels serve as nutrition carriers, e. g., in the epithelium of the skin, cornea of the eye. The lacteal vessels of the intestinal villi have the special function of absorbing the chyle.

The Lymph-glands and their Function.—The function of the lymphatic glands is as yet not fully understood. The glands participate in the production of white blood-cells by the cellular proliferation in the germinal centres, proven by the fact that the lymph is richer in cellular elements after having passed through a chain of glands. A pathological proof of this function is found in leukæmia, the hyperplasia of the lymphatic glands being associated with marked increase of the white blood-cells.

LUCIANI [14] believes that many of the catabolic products poured out by the tissues into the lymph-stream and which, if directly re-absorbed into the blood, would exercise a toxic action, are rendered innocuous by the specific activity of the numerous lymphatic glands through which they pass before joining the blood.

The glands contain a large number of lymphocytes and leucocytes, thus making them of great importance in the organism's fight against infection of any kind.

The anatomical peculiarities of the gland render it a good

filter, whereby many pathogenic bacteria may be arrested or their progress retarded, giving the cellular elements a better chance to attack the invaders.

The glands undergo marked changes during the life of an individual; they are in their fullest stage of development in childhood; and as age advances they become less resilient, the connective tissue increasing in amount, making them less adaptable for filters.

Internal secretion is often spoken of with regard to the lymph-glands, especially the tonsils; but nothing has, as yet, been proven in this respect.

CHAPTER IV

ETIOLOGY

HISTORY

Before the discovery of the Bacillus tuberculosis of KOCH, the etiological conception of enlarged glands, especially of those of the neck, was very vague. The old name, scrofula, often included a variety of conditions such as syphilis, goitre, carcinoma, rickets, etc. Struma was often used in the same sense.

In the early part of the nineteenth century many investigators tried to establish a relationship between scrofula and tuberculosis. The first attempts were followed by negative results. VILLEMIN [1] (1868) succeeded in demonstrating the infectiousness of tuberculosis. He fed dogs with tuberculous lung tissue and thus produced the disease. He also injected substance from caseating lymph glands into two guinea-pigs with positive results. But VILLEMIN'S views were not generally accepted. It remained for ROBERT KOCH to demonstrate and isolate the Bacillus tuberculosis (1882). He proved that the so-called scrofulous glands were tuberculous in nature. KOCH found the tubercle bacilli in a number of glands, which histologically were proven to be tuberculous; animal injections were also followed by positive results.

BACTERIOLOGY

BACILLUS TUBERCULOSIS HUMANUS

Morphology.—The Tubercle Bacillus is a minute rod-shaped organism with slightly rounded ends and a somewhat bent shape. It varies in length from 1.5 to 3.5 microns and in thickness from 0.2 to 0.5 microns. The bacilli occur singly or in groups, often overlapping each other. A marked similarity to the actinomyces is often shown by the appearance of bizarre forms with projecting processes or branches, or club-shaped or beaded organisms. Metachromatic bodies of highly refractile power are often found in the bacilli, giving them a beaded appearance. At first these were thought to be spores but have since been recognized as vacuoles. The tubercle bacillus has no power of movement and does not possess any flagellæ.

Staining Characteristics.—The tubercle bacillus does not stain well with ordinary methods. Koch found that the dye must contain a mordant before it takes. He used a solution of caustic potash to fix the stain. This method was later modified by Ehrlich who found that pure anilin was a better mordant than potash. A still later modification is that of Ziehl-Nielson where carbol-fuchsin is used. The specific staining reaction of tubercle bacillus is that the color once assumed, is both acid and alcohol fast

Much [2] discovered that in tuberculous tissue, especially of bovine origin, where no tubercle bacilli are demonstrable by the Ziehl method, an organism is present which can be stained by Gram's method. A granular form, Much's granules, can also be demonstrated in many cases. The real significance of this granular form is not known. Much and Deycke consider them as the primitive original form, from which the acid-fast tubercle bacilli have developed Much succeeded in changing the non-acid fast type to the acid fast by passing through a guinea-pig. Many investigators believe that they represent products of disintegration. (v. Behring, Cornet, Geipel.) According to the more recent investigations of Bittrolf and Momose, [3] no other form of the tubercle bacillus can be demonstrated by Much's method than by Ziehl's, provided the twenty-four hour method is employed.

Culture Characteristics.—The tubercle bacillus is a strict aerobic organism, requiring considerable oxygen for its growth and therefore grows only upon the surface of the culture-media. The optimum temperature is 37° C., while the temperature below 29° C or above 42° C. inhibit its growth.

Culture on Blood Serum.—Koch was the first to use blood serum as a culture medium; he succeeded by its use in artificially cultivating the organism. In about two weeks the growth is visible to the naked eye, in the form of dry, whitish flakes which increase in size at the edges and form small scale-like masses with a wrinkled surface; the layer is dry and brittle, pushing itself up the side of the tube. Blood serum is useful in isolating fresh virulent cultures.

Culture on Glycerin Agar.—Any of the ordinary culture media will grow the tubercle bacillus, if glycerin is added in amounts of 3 to 5%. Glycerin agar gives a quite luxuriant growth of the organism, resembling that upon the blood serum.

Cultures on Glycerin Bouillon.—A Glycerin Bouillon of acid reaction forms a good medium for the growth of tubercle bacilli, the organisms growing quite rapidly on its surface. A wrinkled crust is formed which gradually becomes thicker and covered with light yellow puffy masses and folds, while the bouillon underneath remains clear.

Resistance to Heat.—If the tubercle bacillus is exposed to moist heat of 55° C. for a period of six hours it is killed; dry heat is borne better. According to SCHILL and FISCHER [4] it can be exposed to a temperature of 100° C. for an hour without being killed.

Pasteurization of milk is a question of marked practical importance. The heating of milk up to 65–70° C. in open vessels is not sufficient for complete sterilization, because the bacteria rise to the top where the temperature is lower. To insure complete pasteurization, the milk has to be stirred or treated in closed vessels. If the latter method is employed good results are obtained by maintaining a temperature of 65° C. for 20 minutes.

Effect of Cold.—Generally speaking, cold does not seem to have any effect on the tubercle bacillus with the exception that the alternate exposure of the organism to thawing and freezing is destructive to its virulence.

Effect of Moisture.—The absence of moisture in the culture tends to decrease the life of the organism. Under ordinary circumstances the culture may retain its virulence for six to eight months. The virulence of sputum is a question of paramount importance. A number of external conditions influence the vitality of the germ, namely, exposure to light, heat and air. Under favorable conditions the tubercle bacilli in dried sputum may retain their vitality for many months.

Action of Light.—Sunlight is the arch enemy of tubercle bacillus. KOCH showed that cultures in thin layers were sterilized within a few minutes when exposed to strong sunlight, while diffused daylight required several days. The combined effect of sunlight and air, without doubt, rapidly destroys the virulence of the tuberculous sputum, even the electric arc light has been proven to have án injurious effect on the bacilli BANGS [5] of the Finsen Light Institute, showed that tuberculous cultures were sterilized after an exposure of from 3 to 9 minutes to this light.

Water as a Harbinger.—Pure water may harbor virulent bacilli for many months under favorable conditions, but in natural conditions the germs are rendered avirulent in a comparatively short time by the effect of light and processes of decomposition.

Action of the Gastric Juice.—The Gastric Juices are inimical to the growth of the tubercle bacilli and may in the test tube even cause their death, but the effect in the human stomach most probably does not play any rôle on account of the varying acid strength of the gastric juice and the short time the food remains there.

Effect of Antiseptics.—The ordinary bactericidal agents such as mercuric chloride, phenol, etc., have very little effect on the tubercle bacilli. A five per cent solution of phenol requires 24 hours to sterilize a culture. But substances having solvent action, such as combinations of soap and the kresols, are very effective. Lysol, for instance, in one per cent solution will kill the bacilli in a comparatively short time. The strongly oxidizing agents are also of value. Calcium hypochlorite is the disinfectant par excellence for sputum and feces.

Chemistry of the Tubercle Bacillus.—The Bacillary Bodies contain substances soluble in alcohol and ether solvents, which consist of fatty acids, neutral fat and wax, also albuminous bodies, carbohydrates and mineral constituents. The amount of fat may reach forty per cent. KLEBS [6] isolated two fatty bodies, one soluble in ether and one in benzine. According to DEYCKE, it is the neutral fats which are responsible for the acid and alcohol resisting power of the bacilli, while the fatty acids give them their specific staining property. The nucleo-proteids extracted by WEIL and H. HOFFMAN and identified by DESCHWEINITZ were analyzed by LEVENE and RUPPEL independently, who succeeded in liberating free nucleinic acid. RUPPEL [7] further succeeded in decomposing this acid into thymin and a neutral substance called "tuberculosin."

Varieties of Tubercle Bacilli.—A great number of color-fast bacilli exist in nature. Of these at least four types belonging to the tubercle bacillus group are pathogenic—namely, the human, bovine, avian and piscine types.

THE BACILLUS TUBERCULOSIS BOVIS.

Morphology.—The bovine bacilli are shorter and thicker than the human type; they are straighter in outline and often somewhat wedge-shaped.

Staining Characteristics.—The Bovine type has the same staining properties as the human type, but as a rule stains more homogeneously and becomes more highly colored.

Culture Characteristics.—The bovine bacillus is more difficult to cultivate, growing more slowly than the human type. According to THEOBALD SMITH it produces an alkaline reaction in broth.

Pathogenesis.—The main differentiating point between bovine and human tubercle bacilli is the difference in their virulence for animals. The human type does not cause progressive tuberculosis in the rabbit; in subcutaneous injection a transitory swelling of the nearest gland may be noticed, but this soon involutes. The bovine type, on the other hand, causes a marked enlargement of the regional glands in three to four weeks; progressive tuberculosis develops, especially in lungs, kidneys, spleen and liver. The human type is nearly non-pathogenic for cattle while the bovine type is highly virulent. The guinea-pig is highly susceptible to both types, although it dies somewhat more quickly from bovine infection.

The Bacillus Tuberculosis Avium.

Morphology.—The Avian tubercle bacillus resembles the human type but fragmental and beaded forms are more common. In staining properties it does not differ from the other types, being both acid and alcohol fast.

Culture Characteristics.—The Avian Bacillus is the least difficult to cultivate. It grows luxuriantly on all culture media; no addition of glycerin is needed for its growth. The culture has a moist creamy consistency, thus differing from the dry appearance of the other types. In contradistinction to the human and bovine types, it retains its virulence when growing at 43° C.

Pathogenesis.—Birds are the most susceptible animals; guinea-pigs are quite immune, but rabbits are easily infected.

The Bacillus Tuberculosis Piscium.

The Reptilian or Piscine type grows readily at low temperature (20°–25° C.). It is not infectious to mammals or birds.

Saprophytic Acid-fast Bacilli.—A number of saprophytic acid-proof bacilli have been described resembling the tubercle bacillus in morphology and staining. The most common are Bacillus smegmatis, Moeller's grass bacillus, butter bacillus of Rabinowitsch and the pseudo-bovine bacillus. They all grow luxuriantly on artificial media and exhibit more often actinomyces-like forms.

Animal inoculation may sometimes lead to production of nodular lesions resembling the tubercles; but they are not caused by the pathogenetic action of the bacilli, but result from the foreign body action.

Phylogenesis and Change of Type.—McFarland states that it is not impossible that the bacilli of human, bovine and avian tuberculosis are closely related to one another and, together with a few other microörganisms of similar morphology and staining peculiarities, have a common ancestry and are descended from the same original stock.

Chabas [8] quoting Ferran says that the acid-fast bacillus of Koch is not the most liable or frequent factor in spreading tuberculosis, because it is impossible by means of this bacillus to explain the enormous incidence of tuberculosis, also other problems in the etiology; the primary changes are due to a group of tuberculogenous, non-acid fast bacteria, which produce an inflammation that can kill in a few hours, or pass into a chronic state producing tubercles, the causative factor, changing into the acid-fast bacillus of Koch.

Much's Granules.—The significance of the so-called Much's granules is not quite known; Much and Deycke consider them the primitive form, from which the typical tubercle bacilli develop, hence playing the same rôle as Ferran's bacteria.

That a biologic relationship [9] exists between the true tubercle bacilli and the non-pathogenic type, is shown by the experiment of Krause who demonstrated that extracts of smegma and grass bacilli are capable of producing tuberculin reactions; Koch also showed that specific tuberculous agglutinating serum caused agglutination of grass bacilli and precipitation of their culture fluid

Relation between Human and Bovine Types.—The relationship between the human and bovine tubercle bacilli is a very hotly disputed question For a number of years after Koch's discovery, the two were considered to be identical. In 1896, Theobald Smith [10] published the results of his exhaustive studies on this particular point. His observations form the foundation for our present knowledge of the differences between the two bacilli. Koch also took up this question, and at the International Congress on Tuberculosis in London (1901) expressed his belief that the human and bovine forms of tuberculosis were caused by different types, if not different species. Various writers have expressed the opinion that the two bacilli are of one and the same species, the apparent differences being due to adaptation to different surroundings; a number of investigators have reported successful attempts to increase the virulence of the human bacillus by passing them through goats. (v. Behring, Pearson, Eber, De Jong, Damman and Muessem-

BLER)—others report negative results (KOSSEL, WEVER, HEUSE, and THEOBALD SMITH.)

Change in Type.—CORNET [11] emphatically denies any possibility for a change from one type to the other, charging every investigator who has succeeded in demonstrating that under certain conditions this very thing may take place, with some fault in the technic. THEOBALD SMITH, L. RABINOWITSCH and DUVAL [12] report the existence of intermediate forms.

v. BEHRING [13] rightly calls attention to the fact that the anthrax bacillus can be changed to a non-sporagenous bacillus and less gradually to an avirulent one. Taking all evidence into consideration, for and against, it must be admitted that conclusive proof is wanting of an actual or permanent transformation of one type into another by the passage through animals, or by culture, but on the other hand, the impossibility of such a change is neither proven.

INCIDENCE OF INFECTION.

The Human Tubercle Bacillus undoubtedly is the most common factor in producing tuberculosis in man. The tubercle bacillus is commonly referred to as ubiquitous, but always with the reservation that it does not multiply outside the animal body. But modern investigations seem to disprove this idea of ubiquity. CORNET [14] showed by exhaustive experiments that the only place where bacilli were found in numbers worth mentioning was in shut-up rooms occupied by tuberculous patients.

The Bovine Type.—The significance of bovine infection in man is an unsettled question. The most opposed views have been put forth. v. Behring's original theory that all tuberculosis is due to the bovine infection acquired in infancy is, at present, considered more or less obsolete by most authors. The opposite opinion, that bovine infection can be ignored, has had many supporters. The exhaustive researches on this particular point during the last few years have enabled us to get a better understanding of this important question. The bovine bacillus has been found time and again to be the causative factor of tuberculous processes in man. While the danger from this source has been exaggerated, it is now proven without any doubt to be a distinct menace.

THEOBALD SMITH, one of the first investigators to differentiate between the human and bovine types of the bacilli (1896) stated that bovine tuberculosis might, under certain conditions, be transmitted to children. KOCH at the British Congress on Tuberculosis (1901) seemed to prove that transmission of the bovine type to man was a very rare occurrence and hence deemed it not advisable to take any measures against it.

Pulmonary tuberculosis in man is, undoubtedly, in the vast majority of cases caused by the human type of bacillus; but researches have disclosed the fact that not a mean percentage of glandular tuberculosis, especially mesenteric and cervical, is caused by the bovine bacillus.

PARK [15] made a very thorough investigation to ascertain the frequency of human tuberculosis in New York City due to bovine tuberculosis; he came to the following conclusion: "Fatal tuberculosis due to bovine bacillus is rare in those over five years of age, but on the other hand, infection of the lymph-nodes is frequent, 30% or more of tuberculous lymph-nodes occurring in children between five and sixteen years of age are contracted through bovine bacilli." Including the result of his own investigation, which involved nearly 500 cases, PARK reports the following cases from the literature:

PARK'S TABLE

DIAGNOSIS	ADULTS 16 yrs.& over Human	Bovine	CHILDREN 5–16 yrs. Human	Bovine	CHILDREN Under 5 yrs. Human	Bovine
Pulmonary Tuberculosis	778	3	14		35	1
Tuberculous Adenitis inguinal or axillary	3		4		2	
Cervical Tuberculosis	36	1	36	22	15	24
Abdominal Tuberculosis	16	4	8	9	10	14
Generalized Tuberculosis, alimentary origin	6	1	3	4	17	15
Generalized Tuberculosis,	29		5	1	74	7
Generalized Tuberculosis, including meninges, alimentary origin			1		5	10
Generalized Tuberculosis, including meninges	5		10		76	1
Tuberculosis of Bones and Joints	32	1	41	3	27	4
Tuberculous Meningitis	1		3		28	
Genito-Urinary Tuberculosis	22	1	2			
Tuberculosis of Tonsils				1		
Tuberculosis of Skin	10	3	4	6	2	
Miscellaneous cases of Tuberculosis						
Tuberculosis of Mouth and Cervical Nodes		1				
Tuberculous sinus or abscess	2					
Septic. Latent bacilli					1	
TOTALS	940	15	131	46	292	76

A. P. MITCHELL [16] considers the part played by the bovine bacillus in the causation of tuberculosis in man, one of the most important public health questions. In post-mortem examinations of 29 cases under 12 years of age he isolated cultures from 12, finding the bovine type in four, and the human in seven cases. The bovine infection represented primary disease of the mesenteric glands, the other primary disease of the bronchial glands in six cases, one being uncertain. Amongst 80 cases of tuberculous cervical glands the same investigator found 71 cases, i. e., 88% due to bovine infection, and 9 to the human type of the bacillus.

Bovine Type Frequent Cause of Tuberculous Lymphadenitis.—
In a recent article MITCHELL [16] again emphasizes the importance
of the bovine bacillus in infection of the tonsil with subsequent
changes in the cervical glands. In 106 cases of distinct tuberculosis of the cervical glands the tonsils on microscopic examination were found to be tuberculous in 38%. Animal inoculation in 92 cases gave 20 positive results, the bovine type of
bacillus being isolated in 16. In 100 cases of hypertrophied
tonsils with barely palpable cervical glands, the tonsils were,
on microscopic examination, found to be tuberculous in 9%.
Animal inoculation gave positive results in all cases, 4 of which
were proven to be bovine in type, 2 human and 3 not determined.

WOODHEAD [17] reports 29 cases of primary abdominal tuberculosis; of these 14 yielded bovine bacilli only, whilst in two
cases both types of bacilli were demonstrated and separated.
Of the 14 cases containing bovine bacilli, 10 were children between the ages of one and three years, 3 between four and five
years and one eight years of age. From these observations it is
clearly seen that the bovine tubercle bacillus plays a very definite
rôle in production of tuberculous lesions during childhood,
especially those of the abdominal organs and cervical glands.
Both of these forms of tuberculosis are often due to ingestion of
tuberculous infective material. A nearly universal diet for
children is milk; hence it is seen what an important rôle milk
plays in transferring the bovine bacillus upon the human host.

SOURCE OF INFECTION

Cow's milk is, without question, the most common medium
by which bovine tuberculosis is transferred to man. BANGS in
Denmark was the first investigator to emphasize the importance
of a rigid milk inspection. Examination of the milk supply has
been made in a number of cities, and it shows that raw market
milk of the cheaper grades in most cities frequently contains
bovine tubercle bacilli. PARK examined 100 samples of milk
in New York (1908) and found 12% infected; in 1912 he found
6%. In examination of Edinburgh's supply of milk (406 samples)
MITCHELL found 20% were tuberculous.

How does the milk become infected? The most common mode is by the presence of a tuberculous udder. In these cases the milk may contain an enormous number of bacilli. These ulcers of the udder are sometimes so small that they cannot be noticed with the naked eye; but an open ulcer of the udder is not required to infect the milk.

The tuberculous cow may cough, swallow the bacilli and pass them with the feces. Contamination of the milk may thus easily occur, especially on the average farm where ideas of hygiene and cleanliness are not what they ought to be.

Tuberculous meat, beef or pork, most probably is not of very great consequence. Meat, as a rule, is quite thoroughly cooked before it is consumed, hence if any bacilli should happen to be present the chances are that they would be killed; on the other hand, meat forms a comparatively small part in the diet of children who, as has been demonstrated, are most susceptible to bovine infection.

OTHER FACTORS HAVING BEARING ON THE ETIOLOGY

Predisposition.—The fatalistic theory of a specific predisposition to tuberculosis has had for centuries a stranglehold upon the human mind. Even during later years theories have been advanced and constitutions described tending to prove the positive existence of such a condition. Hippocrates described a "habitus phthisicus" which does not differ very much from the tuberculous habitus described by modern authors. But all these cases of predisposition undoubtedly represent the first stages of the disease. Modern investigations have disclosed the fact that nearly all human beings have, or have had, a tuberculous infection. Hence, it would seem that nearly all are predisposed. It is consequently irrational to speak of a predisposition to tuberculosis in a certain few when the greatest majority of the human family, at least those in touch with civilization, have been proven to be attacked.

The subsequent development of the disease is another matter depending upon entirely other factors, viz.:—massiveness of the infection, virulence of the bacilli, resistance of the individual—not to be confused with predisposition—age when attacked, time of diagnosis and treatment of the disease. If we speak of predisposition to tuberculosis in the broadest sense of the word, viz.:—comparing the effect on different races, we may have some excuse for using the term. But even here, there is a chance for argument. Many races were for a long time considered immune to the disease, but later happenings indicated that they had not been exposed before, because as a result of closer contact with civilization—hence with infection—they soon were ravished by a severe form of the disease. But the lack of natural immunity is quite different from predisposition.

The fact that the civilized races are not the victims of such severe forms of the disease proves that something entirely opposed to predisposition exists, viz.:—a resistance which tends to lessen the virulence of the disease, an acquired racial immunity. Several races have been said to be particularly resistant to the disease: the Jewish race for instance, whose manner of living, social conditions, city life, etc., have certainly given this people a resistance which, under ordinary conditions, would prove and does prove to be of great value. But look at the congested districts of the greater cities often inhabited only by Jews. Is not tuberculosis common among them? Consider the Chinese as found in America. The mortality from tuberculosis amongst them does not differ very much from that of the negro. The resistance of the ancient Chinese race against tuberculosis gained from contact with the disease for thousands of years is not great enough to overcome the depreciating effects of unhygienic living, excessive labor and many vices common amongst so many of the Chinese in this country.

Hereditary Predisposition.—This ancient supposition, investigated at a time when the real nature of the disease was not known, still plays quite an important rôle according to some authors in propagation of the disease; the great mass of people believe it, and the family of the tuberculous person regards it with horror. The theory is based on the well-known fact that children of tuberculous parents develop tuberculosis quite frequently. Before the infectious nature of the disease was known this theory explained many more or less obscure facts.

The hereditary predisposition gave a perfect explanation why so many in the same family succumbed to the disease. But it has also removed the hope from many individuals who, under normal conditions, would be able to fight the affection with success. It is impossible to estimate how many lives have been ended prematurely, on account of this fatalistic teaching; the stricken patient was absolutely convinced that he did not have any chance whatsoever in the struggle for life, and hence fell an easy prey to this illness which, bar none, requires the most optimistic state of mind for success in its treatment.

It is true that tuberculosis often is a family disease, but not on account of any hereditary tendency, but on account of the increased opportunities of infection due to close contact in the ordinary family life. That this is true is proven by the fact that if the baby is removed from the tuberculous surroundings and protected from the ordinary opportunities of infection, he will remain healthy in the great majority of instances.

Previous Diseases.—The acute infectious diseases certainly play some rôle in awakening a previously dormant tuberculous focus to activity. We often have latent inactive foci in the lymphatics In childhood the lymphatic glands are very sensitive to tuberculous infection. It is common to find tuberculosis following many of the acute or wasting diseases of childhood, and the infection seems to show a predilection for the lymphnodes. Considering the enormous morbidity of measles, whooping cough and influenza, COPELAND [18] thinks that the incidence of tuberculosis, as a complication or sequela, is of relatively importance

GANGHOFNER [19] of Prague gives the following table to show the incidence of the tuberculous infection in acute infectious diseases:

Heller of Kiel—714 cases dead from acute infectious
diseases—140 tuberculous or 19 6%
Councilman of Boston—220 cases—35 tuberculous, 16%
Baginsky of Berlin   806   "   144   "   17 8%
Ganghofner of Prague 973   "   253   "   28%

v. Pirquet has shown that there is an allergic reaction
during the first stage of measles. Rolly has proven that the
same thing is true in pneumonia, scarlet fever and severe constitutional diseases. The acute infections are characterized by
a marked catarrhal inflammation of the mucous membranes over
the entire body, and by greatly lowered resistance, also attended
with intense hyperemia and lymphatic activity. If there are
any latent foci of tuberculosis in the body the increased vascular
changes will cause the bacilli to penetrate the zones of infiltration
and settle in different places of the body. The lymph-glands are
the most likely to be affected on account of their lessened resistance caused by repeated attacks of infectious diseases—
measles, whooping cough, influenza and catarrhal infections.
The lowered general resistance of the body to tuberculosis
shown by the allergic tuberculin reaction gives the tuberculous
infection a chance to progress.

Nervous System.—Changes in the nervous system manifested
by instability, as exhibited in the children of neurotic, neurasthenic parents, constitute no mean part in our etiologic picture.
Often nervous affections are found in certain families and are
known to alternate between tuberculous parent and offspring.
Thus, for instance, in a tuberculous family you will see one of
the children dying of tuberculous meningitis, another developing
tuberculous lymphadenitis, while the third may escape the
diathesis but become a neurotic.

Alcohol is an important predisposing factor as exhibited in
the children of alcoholic parents. They are weak in body, sub-
normals morally and mentally, and fall an easy prey to tuberculous infections.

Digestive disturbances in children lower their resistance and
on account of the inflammatory condition of the intestinal mucous
membrane facilitate the intrusion of the tubercle bacilli, hence
causing infection of the mesenteric glands. Young [20] examined a
number of children suffering from apparent malnutrition but
with no sign, symptom or history of tuberculosis. The v. Pirquet
test gave the following results:

55 children under 1 year, 7 positive, 12.7%
85   "   " 1½ " 15   "   18.2%
93   "   " 2 " 19   "   20.4%

Under-feeding of high grade undoubtedly has a pronounced bearing upon the resistance to any disease. But it is especially tuberculosis that watches its chances carefully and gets a foot-hold whenever the vigilance of the defensive mechanism of the body is slackened.

Malnutrition constitutes one of the most important factors in exposing the child to tuberculous infection. These underfed, poorly nourished children are especially subject to frequent colds, nasal catarrh, respiratory tract defects. They are anæmic, fretful, peevish, selfish and difficult to manage.

Repeated infections of the upper air passages, so common every fall and spring, have a deleterious effect upon the lymphatic apparatus of the neck; the lymphatic glands become less and less capable to cope with the infections. If a few tubercle bacilli should make their appearance, the lymphoid tissue would not have enough resisting power to ward off their attack and prevent their propagation and the subsequent changes.

Disease of the tonsils and adenoids decreases the resisting power of the organism and renders these organs more susceptible to tuberculous infection. Their rôle in actual infection will be taken up in a later chapter.

Dental defects have not received the attention they are entitled to in the genesis of tuberculosis, and also other diseases. For the first six months of life, the mucous membrane of the mouth is continuous and intact, but after that period hard structures pierce through its external surface, and continue to do so, by a process termed eruption of teeth until adult life. Under normal conditions the child erupts at six months two incisor teeth, and completes the eruption of twenty teeth before three years.

Physiologically these deciduous teeth should not decay, but under the influence of the child's greater activity, biting and chewing, associated with the pressure from below of the permanent teeth, they should spread apart, loosen at their roots, fall out and be immediately replaced with their permanent successors.

Even under normal conditions the functions of the lymphatic apparatus is markedly taxed during these physiological changes. But how much more work is thrown upon it when decay of the teeth sets in.

Dental caries, the most common of all diseases, transform the teeth into regular cesspools of infection. This constant absorption of toxins from the dental cavities must undoubtedly set its stamp upon the lymphatic glands concerned in their drainage, and lower their resistance in a marked degree. The transmission of the tubercle bacilli will be discussed in the chapter dealing with portals of entry.

Pedley's Views.—PEDLEY [21] says that the inability to masticate food in order to prepare it properly for gastric digestion, the constant nervous irritation caused by the exposure of one pulp-chamber after another, the accumulation of putrid and decomposing material in cavities already the home of innumerable bacteria, with the vitiated secretions, are in themselves sufficient to produce in the growing child a lowered vitality which renders it a ready prey to other disorders of the body.

Environments. The Influence of Climate and Topography.— The old ideas that certain regions of the earth were free from tuberculosis on account of some inherent property and that some regions were especially conducive to it, are not longer held. The different places considered to be immune to tuberculosis, are now proven to have been simply uninfected territory. But as BALDWIN [22] expresses it, "The debilitating heat of the tropics, with the high humidity, and the depressing effects of the fogs and wet winds of the Atlantic coast, must only be contrasted with the invigorating highlands of the interior, and the arid deserts and sunny tablelands of the far west, to admit that climate is a potent factor in physiological resistance to tuberculosis."

The social conditions undoubtedly have a pronounced bearing upon the development of tuberculosis in all its forms. Tuberculosis is mainly a disease of the poor, the overworked, the underpaid, the underfed, although the more prosperous members of society have to contribute their share. Unhygienic living conditions is the one single factor which, next to the actual presence of the causative germ, determines the propagation of this disease.

The Home an Important Factor.—Tuberculosis has often been called a house disease, and that rightly. It is the careless consumptive in the home who is the most potent factor in spreading this disease. The tuberculous father, mother, sister or brother, expectorates indiscriminately, is not overly clean in his or her habits, fondles and kisses the innocent baby.

The greater importance of the droplet infection or that by dried sputum is an academic question which in practice can be overlooked. They are both of marked importance. The bacillus preserves its virulence long enough in both the dry and wet state to be dangerous.

The tuberculous individual may cough in the face of the child, or expectorate on the floor—the baby's playground—the effect is the same. The bacilli are bound to be introduced into the highly susceptible body of the young child.

Crowded dwellings with dark rooms in which the sun scarcely enters and where ventilation is an unheard of thing, are veritable breeding places of tuberculosis. Granted one of these houses and an individual with open tuberculosis, not overly careful, what chance have the children in that household? ABSOLUTELY NONE—they all become infected. How many families live, or rather try to exist, in damp, musty cellar dwellings? Lack of all conception of personal hygiene certainly is responsible for a great number of cases; uncleanliness in dwellings permits the accumulation of bacteria and hence increases the chances of infection; lack of care of the skin favors the retention of any bacteria with which the individual has come in contact; pediculosis, according to some authors, plays a definite rôle in production of tuberculous cervical adenitis. What value will ultimately be assigned to casual infection such as occurs through the agency of street dust, flies, water and fomites is hard to tell; at present there is a tendency to believe that direct, intense and prolonged contact is necessary for infection.

Schools.—The contact in school is hardly of intimate enough character to be conducive of infection. Open tuberculosis is quite rare in children and hence it is out of the question to transmit the disease from child to child. The schoolmaster with productive lesions certainly is a distinct menace to the pupils and should be guarded against.

Factory.—The unsanitary, poorly lighted, scantily heated and ill-ventilated factory or shop employing a large amount of child-labor certainly plays its rôle in the production and spreading of this disease. The report of the investigation made by the U. S. Commissioner of Labor [23] into the conditions surrounding working women and children shows that of the employees in the cotton textile industry 5.2% in the northern mills, and 20% in the southern mills are children under sixteen. In North and South Carolina, thirty mills employed 549 children from eleven and one-half to twelve hours a night for five nights in the week. The same report referring to mortality among cotton mill operatives shows that the child who works in a cotton mill has only half as good a chance to live to be 20 years old as the child outside the mill, and the 1910 census reports 41,000 child operatives in the cotton mills of the country. Among the cotton mill operatives approximately one of every two deaths between fifteen and forty-four years of age was found to be due to tuberculosis.

The Frequency with which Tuberculosis is Found in Childhood

At the present time there is a very strong tendency to believe that nearly all cases of tuberculosis have had their origin in early childhood. Proofs for this supposition are not lacking. The cutaneous tuberculin reaction, so rare during the first few months of life, increases in frequency with every year, to reach its height between the ages of 10 and 15 years.

Children are Born Free from Tuberculosis.—Children are, on the whole, born free from tuberculosis; ten per cent are infected at the end of the first year, and only ten per cent free at sixteen years of age.

The following table gives the findings of various investigators: [24]

Name	Number of children tested	Age at which largest percentage of positive reactions are obtained	Percentage of reactions
v. Pirquet	1407	13–14	93%
Hamburger	532	13–15	95%
Hellesen	480	10–14	46%
Shaw & Baird	330	over 6	45%
Meroz & Khalatoff	337	10–15	78.8%
McNeil	541	4–15	45%
Berberich	800	10–15	58.8%
Lapage	1000	5–10	68.8%
Arieti	38	7–11	59%
Fishberg	692	14	83.9%
Fishberg	588	14	75%
Veeder & Johnson	1321	10–14	44%
Manning & Knott	228	10–14	58.1%
Rosquist	472	14–15	76.5%

Different Results Obtained.—The difference in results obtained by various observers cannot be easily explained; some authors believe that the discrepancies must be attributed to differences of technic; but MANNING [25] is of the opinion that the peculiarities of climate, sanitation and housing of the different communities are responsible for the different results. Undoubtedly there is some difference in the prevalence of tuberculosis in the poorer districts of Vienna and New York, and the smaller towns of Western America.

Observers in larger cities find comparatively small difference between the frequency of tuberculosis amongst children of tuberculous and those of non-tuberculous parents. FISHBERG'S [26] findings certainly are expressive; the children in the tenement districts of New York, tuberculosis or no tuberculosis in the family, will in the majority of cases become infected.

FISHBERG'S TABLE

Percentage giving positive reactions among

	Children of tuberculous parents		Children of non-tuberculous parents	
Age	No. of cases	%	No. of cases	%
Under 1 yr.	33	15.15	56	10.07
1–2 years	49	55.10	39	33.33
3–4 "	90	68.88	80	41.25
5–6 "	95	65.26	106	50.
7–10 "	244	71.31	173	64.74
11–14 "	181	74.58	134	69.40
14 "	37	83.79	20	75.

That the opportunity for infection is less in the smaller town is shown by the findings of MANNING and KNOTT.[27] They come to the conclusion that children living in a tuberculous milieu react in ratio of about two to one of those living in an environment not known to be tuberculous.

FINDINGS OF MANNING AND KNOTT

Reactions of Exposed and Non-exposed Children:

	Positive v. Pirquet		Negative v. Pirquet	
166 children exposed	84	50.6%	82	49.3%
62 " with no known exposure	14	22.8%	48	77.4%
228	98	42.9%	130	57.1%

Tuberculosis in Infancy a Severe Affair.—Tuberculosis in early infancy is a very severe affair; the tendency for the disease to become generalized is very marked, and it usually results in death. BROWN[28] made the tuberculin skin test on 650 cases of infants and reports the following findings: of 62 infants between the age of one and three months 13 gave a positive reaction. They all died, and the diagnosis was confirmed by autopsy. Of 102 cases between the ages of three and six months, 7 reacted positively, 6 of those died and the autopsy confirmed the diagnosis. Forty-three positive reactions were found amongst 217 infants between six and twelve months; 35 proved to be tuberculous. Of 156 cases between twelve and seventeen months, 37 gave a positive reaction. Twenty of these proved to be tuberculous by autopsy or bacillary findings, 16 were discharged as improved or cured. One hundred and twelve infants between eighteen months and two years of age were examined, 24 gave a positive reaction, 15 of which proved to be tuberculous by autopsy or bacillary findings, 4 were moribund on admission, and 5 were discharged as improved or cured.

Autopsy Findings.—WOLLSTEIN and BARTLETT [29] report the findings of 1,320 autopsies performed at the Babies Hospital of the city of New York, 178 of which showed tuberculous lesions, i. e., 13.5%. The age varied from 2½ months to five years, 75% of the cases being under two years. The great majority of the cases (75%) were generalized infections with tuberculous lesions involving the lungs and bronchial lymph-nodes, as the most advanced.

LUBARCH [30] found among 747 children up to age of 5 years, 128 cases of tuberculosis, or 17%. ROTHE [31] verified his postmortem examinations on 100 children by inoculating parts of both the bronchial and mesenteric glands into guinea-pigs and gave the following report:

Age	No. examined	Positive results in animal experiments	
		No.	Percentage
0–1 year	49	7	14.3
1–2 "	28	9	32.14
2–3 "	8	2	25.
3–4 "	8	3	37.5
4–5 "	7	0	0
TOTAL	100	21	21.%

TUBERCULOUS INFECTION VS. TUBERCULOUS DISEASE

Taking into consideration the large number of children who react positively to the tuberculin test, MORSE'S [32] distinction between tuberculous infection and tuberculous disease seems rather well taken. He defines infection as the state of being infected and disease as an alteration in the state of the body or of some of its organs, interrupting or disturbing the performance of the vital functions and causing symptoms of some sort. A comparatively small proportion of the children showing a positive v. Pirquet test have tuberculous disease; they are, however, infected. It is the reaction of the tissue to the infection that constitutes the disease tuberculosis; this is also known as clinical tuberculosis.

Children Susceptible to Infection.—The figures above show that children are very susceptible to tuberculous infection and if the disease attacks any other organ but the glands, death usually ensues. Pulmonary tuberculosis is nearly universally fatal in children.

As has been shown by the above figures, tuberculosis increases in frequency with each year during childhood, but it also decreases in fatality; there is some reason to believe that under a certain age resistance to the disease is not developed. WOLLSTEIN and BARTLETT in their series of cases did not encounter one single healed lesion, and attempts at healing, shown by calcified areas, were found only five times in the lungs and 13 times in the lymph-nodes; only twice in infants under one year of age.

Location of Infection in Children.—Post-mortem findings indicate that the most common site of tuberculous lesions in early infancy is in the bronchial and mesenteric glands. In early childhood the cervical glands run a close third. In MEDINS [33] series of 632 tuberculous infants under one year the localization was as follows:

In lungs only	78 cases
In bronchial glands only	17 "
In both lungs and bronchial glands without involvement of the digestive tract	194 "
In intestine and mesenteric glands only	6 "
In portal glands and liver only	1 "
In other organs only	7 "
In respiratory and digestive tract	313 "
Location not given	7 "

In GAFFEY'S [34] 300 cases, inoculation experiments showed the bronchial and mesenteric glands were simultaneously involved in 29 cases; bronchial alone in 17 cases and the mesenteric alone in 11 cases.

In ROTHE'S [35] 100 infants under five years the respective figures were 13, 5 and 3.

WOLLSTEIN and BARTLETT'S [36] series of autopsies on 178 tuberculous children under five years gives the following distribution:

```
Lungs..................................................164
Bronchial glands.......................................169
Mesenteric glands......................................113
Mesenteric glands unaccompanied by bronchial involvement.   9
```

HEDREN [37] performed 690 autopsies on children and found tuberculosis in 47 cases under one year and in 152 cases over one year. He gives the following distribution:

Children under one year:

```
Bronchial lymph-glands...........................100  %
Lungs............................................97.8%
Spleen...........................................82.9%
Liver............................................61.7%
Mesenteric lymph-glands..........................57.4%
Intestines.......................................38.3%
Kidneys..........................................34. %
Meninges and brain...............................36.6%
Cervical lymph-glands............................29.9%
Heart............................................10.6%
Pancreas......................................... 4.2%
Adenoids......................................... 3.1%
Tonsils.......................................... 2.1%
```

Children over one year:

```
Bronchial lymph-glands...........................93.4%
Lungs............................................91.4%
Spleen...........................................68.4%
Liver............................................57.8%
Mesenteric lymph-glands..........................48. %
Intestines.......................................33.6%
Meninges and brain...............................61.8%
Kidneys..........................................27.6%
Cervical lymph-glands............................11.2%
```

With regard to the age incidence in tuberculous cervical adenitis, FISCHER [38] who has collected 1,484 cases gives the following percentage during different ages:

FISCHER'S TABLE

Age	No. of cases	Per cent
1- 5	59	3.97
6-10	120	8.08
11-15	233	15.7
16-20	469	31.6
21-25	282	19.
26-30	130	8.67
31-35	63	7.25
36-40	43	2.89
41-45	25	1.68
46-55	29	1.95
56-65	18	1.21

In the author's series of 270 cases of tuberculous cervical adenitis, the percentage was as follows:

Age	No. of cases	Per cent
1- 5	7	2.58
6-10	34	12.59
11-15	142	52.59
16-20	78	28.88
over 20	9	3.33

These figures show that the frequency of cervical glandular tuberculosis is most marked in the second decade. This undoubtedly is dependent upon the concomitant frequency of decayed teeth and diseased tonsils during the same period. The importance of these avenues of infection will be further discussed under pathogenesis.

THE RELATION BETWEEN SCROFULOSIS AND TUBERCULOSIS

The conception of scrofulosis is not as yet fully understood. A number of opinions have been given as to what the term should include—a number of theories have been advanced in order to explain the underlying factors. Several attempts have been made to divide the truly compact mass of clinical manifestations, described under this term, into simpler entities. The old conception of scrofulosis is purely a clinical one, the principal features of which are the peculiar pasty bloated face, associated with inflammations of the eyes, chronic catarrh of the nasal cavities with discharge, swollen overlip, facial eczema and inflammatory changes in the mucous membranes, coupled with glandular swellings.

After the discovery of the tubercle bacillus, a marked relation was proven to exist between many cases of scrofulosis, so-called, and tuberculosis. The bacillus of KOCH was found in a number of enlarged glands and various skin lesions. These findings then led many to believe that scrofulosis was just a manifestation of tuberculosis. The close relation between the two conditions was further proven when it was shown that a majority of children exhibiting the above picture gave a positive tuberculin reaction. The fact that a certain number of these children gave a negative v. Pirquet test seems to prove that this condition is not always a result of tuberculous infection. This opens the way for a more accurate classification of this symptom complex as will be further shown in the chapter on Tuberculin Diagnosis.

Cornet's Views.—If the old conception of scrofulosis with its variety of manifestations is to be maintained, CORNET's [39] standpoint seems rational. In his masterly treatise on scrofulosis he describes the two types—the pyogenic and the tuberculous, admitting that the latter of these is by far the most common. But he does not believe that the genesis of this condition is sufficiently accounted for by the intrusion of bacilli. CORNET does not take kindly to the theories of general diathesis advanced by several authors, but believes that local peripheral peculiarities, present in youth, are responsible for the development of scrofulosis. He proposes the theory that a difference exists in the permeability of the skin and mucous membranes in youth and older age and amongst different individuals.

The skin and mucous membrane of the child are more permeable than those of the older person. Their lymphatics are larger in size, their glands more complex in development, hence bacteria, CORNET concludes, be they pus cocci or tubercle bacilli, can penetrate easier, irritation phenomena be produced and the picture of scrofulosis finally be completed.

This localized diathesis he calls "embryonalism." CORNET's apparently logical reasoning is not without its faults. His theory of varying permeability of the skin and mucous membrane has not received general recognition, nor has it been anatomically proven. Undoubtedly it is a difficult thing to prove by absolute measurements, but, granted that he is right—which he may be—because there is no reason why the stomata in the skin and mucous membrane should not vary in size just as other structures, and as CORNET points out, the variation has only to be so very minute, why should the infection differ so markedly from an ordinary case of pus infection which, for the sake of argument, we will assume CORNET admits may occur in children?

Let us take the eye; a pneumococcus infection of the eye may be mild or severe, but it never takes on the characteristics of the phlyctenular affection associated with the so-called scrofulous manifestations. It would seem that the effect of the bacterial invasion upon an area of greater permeability would produce a more severe condition than under ordinary circumstances.

That phlyctenular inflammation of the eye is a tuberculous affair has been proven time and time again by the wonderful success with tuberculin treatment in these cases. Then why call this a symptom of scrofulosis when it is a manifestly tuberculous condition? That pyogenic cocci of remarkably low virulence may produce a disease resembling it very much is no reason why the tuberculous entity should be overlooked, and confused under the ambiguous term of scrofulosis. The same is true in a more pronounced degree in regard to the lymphatic glands.

Some authors even go so far as to define scrofula as a synonym for tuberculous adenitis. CORNET, at least, is consistent and calls tuberculosis of any gland in the body a manifestation of scrofulosis. But greater permeability of the skin and mucous membrane, or no greater permeability, tuberculous lymph-glands certainly comprise a distinct clinical entity, be the bronchial, mesenteric, cervical or axillary glands involved. To be sure, there are some which are more or less difficult to differentiate from non-tuberculous enlargements, but this is no reason to combine two different conditions under a common term.

With regard to tuberculosis of bones and joints, CORNET admits that this affection appears independently of scrofulosis in the train of tuberculosis of other organs; but still he speaks of scrofulosis of the bone, describing the tuberculous symptom complex. The old conception of scrofulosis certainly did include the tuberculous affections of bones and joints, but why should this antiquated teaching be perpetuated when there is no reason for its existence? It does not simplify matters, but has rather complicated them.

CORNET believes that the bovine type of the tubercle bacillus forms a very considerable source of scrofulous tuberculosis, especially tuberculosis of the neck and mesenteric glands. In his chapter on prognosis, he expresses it as his fixed opinion that a considerable part of scrofulosis, about one-third, is induced by the bovine bacillus and that this, being a bacillus of foreign species, is the cause of the milder course of this disease, compared with the rapid course of internal tuberculosis in children. Consequently, according to CORNET, 33% of scrofulosis is caused by bovine infection made possible by greater permeability of the skin and mucous membranes, and its comparatively mild course is due to the low virulence of the causative germ. Granted this is true—why call it scrofulosis and not infection with bovine type of the tubercle bacilli? In discussing the other 66% CORNET accepts, to a certain extent, theories of greater resisting power of the glands as explanation for the mild course of scrofulosis.

Virchow's Views.—VIRCHOW's theory of inflammatory diathesis, a condition characterized by constitutional weaknesses of the skin, mucous membranes and lymphatics, forms the foundation for the more modern theories of status lymphaticus and exudative diathesis. Virchow considered the inflammatory diathesis as a marked predisposing factor in the development of scrofulosis, and thought it to be due to maldevelopment of the glands and lymphatics, whereby they were rendered more vulnerable to infection.

Escherich's Theory.—In developing the theory of status lymphaticus, ESCHERICH [40] was mainly considering the rôle played by the lymphatic structures; this author and MORO consider this condition not as a diathesis but as the process itself manifested by inflammatory reactions of obstinate nature.

Scrofulosis, according to their conception, is due to a tuberculous infection developed upon the underlying foundation of this lymphatic state.

Czerny's Theory.—CZERNY [41] developing the theory of exudative diathesis considered the condition of the skin and mucous membrane as the main factor, hence the name. In his attempts to establish an etiology, he differed markedly from other men. He proposed that this condition called by him exudative diathesis was due to a disturbance of the intermediary fat metabolism. A certain defect in the body composition renders the child unable to take care of the same amount of fat as a healthy child. In his conception of exudative diathesis, Czerny includes many phenomena described by others as scrofulosis, e. g., blepharitis, eczematous skin lesions and vesicular eruptions, hence denying the relation between the scrofulous habitus and tuberculous infection. To prove this, Czerny calls attention to the fact that he is able to remove the scrofulous habitus by proper feeding, reducing the amount of fats. HEUBNER substantiates this, but reminds us that the same result may be attained by tuberculin treatment.

Heubner's Views.—HEUBNER [42] considers the scrofulous symptom complex as an expression of an underlying tuberculous infection. As proof for this he gives the following findings. The catarrhal condition of the skin and mucous membrane is preceded or soon followed by glandular tuberculosis. Post-mortem findings indicate that all children with so-called scrofulous habitus have tuberculous bronchial glands. Tuberculous children may suddenly develop scrofulosis. Nearly all scrofulous children show a positive tuberculin reaction.

Salge's Views.—SALGE'S [43] conception of scrofulosis coincides with that of Heubner's. With regard to the more or less hypothetical theories of various diatheses, Salge believes that it is more to the point on account of the close connection proven to exist between scrofula and tuberculosis, to ascribe even the peripheral affections of the former symptoms complex to the latter disease, instead of to something else, which nobody has seen nor proven.

SALGE also urges that we must accustom ourselves to regard the scrofulous individual as infected with tuberculosis, which for the time is quiescent and not dangerous, but is apt at any time to assume such a rôle under favorable conditions; such conditions are unhygienic surroundings and malnutrition.

Hochsinger's Views.—HOCHSINGER [44] does not believe with Escherich that the lymphatic hypertrophy is congenital nor with Czerny that hyperplasia of the adenoid tissue is due to an exudative diathesis caused by faulty feeding, but rather that it is the result of repeated infections of early childhood. Hochsinger considers scrofulosis a disease of hygienic neglect, caused by non-specific infections (pediculosis) in a child who is already tuberculous, hence dependent upon some sort of interreaction between pyogenic and tuberculous infections. Hochsinger believes that the picture thus produced is quite characteristic and well limited and should not, although it stands in intimate relationship with tuberculous infection, be confused with tuberculosis but be called scrofulosis. This author also expresses the opinion that the typically tuberculous lesions of skin, joints and glands should not be included in the scrofulous symptom complex, but be considered as truly tuberculous.

Saltmann's Views.—SALTMANN [45] retaining the old conception of scrofulosis, considers it an hereditary tuberculosis, not due to the actual presence of bacilli but rather of their toxins, which, passing through the placenta, poison the developing organism. The result of such poisoning, he believes, is the cause of the scrofulous constitution with a tendency toward acquiring tuberculosis. This theory presupposes the presence of tuberculous toxins in the circulating blood of the pregnant mother, a condition which is hardly plausible. One thing that speaks strongly against the theory is the fact that the tuberculin reaction is very rarely positive in newborn children, hence rendering it very improbable that tuberculous toxins are present in the body of the newborn.

From the above statements we realize how absolute lack of unity exists with regard to scrofulosis, both as to its etiology and as to what ought to be comprised in the symptom complex.

The tendency to simplify the conception of this disease is seen in Heubner's and Salge's views, according to whom scrofulosis is a peculiar manifestation of tuberculosis.

Eustace Smith's Views.—In this connection it is interesting to note the views expressed by Eustace Smith (London) in his text-book on "Disease in Children": [46]

"Scrofula or struma, described as a widespread constitutional hereditary, obstinate and although allied to and often conjoined with tuberculous manifestations, a perfectly distinct and separate entity, has until recent times occupied a prominent place amongst the diseases of early life. More modern views, however, regard the condition as merely a variety of the tuberculous infections which is strictly localized and runs a slow course; and although, like the acute variety it may involve organs of vital importance to the economy, affords more space for treatment, and is more responsive to remedial measures than the rapid generalized form which never spares, but hurries on relentlessly to its close.

It is now held that whether the complaint move quickly or slowly, it owes its origin to one definite infecting agent, the tubercle bacillus; and it is presumable that the precise shape the disease will take, is dependent upon the particular standard of virulence of the organism and the more or less congenial soil in which its work is carried on. The strumous disposition was understood to show itself, especially in glandular enlargements, caseation and softening, chronic erosions and suppurations of bone, obstinate ulcerations of the skin, and other such slowly advancing lesions; but these changes are now recognized as local tuberculous infections due to the entrance into the body of the special bacillus."

The American ideas on scrofulosis vary markedly. HOLT [47] in his text-book on "Diseases in Infancy and Childhood" remarks in discussing the subject of lymphatic diathesis with its tendency to swellings and hyperplasia of the lymphatic structures, that this was formerly classed as one of the manifestations of scrofula, or struma, and that the proof that most of the manifestations, once called scrofulous, are really forms of tuberculosis, makes it undesirable to use that term to designate the condition under discussion. When treating the subject of tuberculous adenitis, HOLT gives it the synonym scrofula; hence being absolutely opposed in his views to those of BALDWIN [48] who says that the much disputed term, scrofula, deserves retention only when applied to chronic non-tuberculous enlargements of the lymph-nodes, and to constitutional weakness of the skin and lymphatic apparatus (inflammatory diathesis) described by Virchow.

The author urges that the name scrofula be discontinued, thus eliminating the confusion which has existed because of the inclusion of several conditions under this term. Exudation or inflammatory diathesis is a distinct condition in itself and when found with tuberculous adenitis it has undoubtedly played the part of a predisposing factor. But the tuberculous adenitis should be recognized as tuberculous and treated as such. In my experience I have found that the vast majority of chronic glandular enlargements, excluding such conditions as Hodgkin's disease and syphilis, were tuberculous in origin rather than due to simple infection.

From this discussion it seems apparent that the old conception of scrofulosis, clinical as it was, included a variety of manifestations which etiologically did not belong to each other. The conditions described as inflammatory diathesis, lymphatism, lymphatic diathesis, exudative diathesis undoubtedly have something in common. It may be some fundamental disturbance in the lymphatic apparatus, or it may be some abnormal state in the chemical composition, or metabolic changes of the organism which are responsible for the same, the fact remains. At present it stands in no relation to scrofulosis so-called, with the exception that the general resistance may be lowered and hence render the child an easier victim to infection. That scrofulosis in some way was dependent upon a tuberculous infection has been the opinion of most authors. The so-called scrofulous glands have been proven to be tuberculous, if we exclude CORNET'S pyogenic variety, but even if the differentiation between these two conditions is difficult, their being different entities cannot be denied, then why include them under the same name? The individuality of the phlyctenular eye lesions, lupus, bone and joint lesions, have already been discussed. Hence it seems advisable to discontinue the use of the term scrofulosis and replace it with tuberculosis when the condition is tuberculous, pyogenic infection when pus cocci are the cause, or a manifestation of exudative or lymphatic diathesis when no more definite etiological factor can be determined.

CHAPTER V

PATHOLOGY

Pathogenesis

In discussing the pathogenesis of tuberculosis, we are entering upon a subject which, during recent years, has received marked attention. In spite of the enormous amount of study and investigation, opinions are still divided as to the most common modes of infection.

Modes of Infection.—That infection occurs in childhood, seems to be nearly universally accepted, and also that the lymphatic apparatus is most commonly affected—but opinions as to the avenues of infection differ markedly. v. Baumgarten is a strong believer in the congenital transmission of the disease, v. Behring and Calmette in the enterogenous mode of infection, but the great majority of authors and investigators hold to the bronchogenous mode of infection. Experimental and clinical proof exist that infection may take place through any of these routes, but the comparative frequency of each one is the difficult thing to estimate.

Infection Through Infected Ovum or Semen. Congenital Transmission.—A number of experiments have been made in order to ascertain the possibility of such an infection. The majority of investigators have had negative results. A few have succeeded in finding the bacilli in embryo after infection of the seminal fluid, but these experiments were made under conditions far removed from those existing in nature. Hence, we must agree with Calmette [1] that no absolute proofs exist that the father can directly transmit the infection.

Direct hereditary transmission from the mother may be possible, but, if so, it is very rare because as Virchow [2] has observed, an ovum infected with tubercle bacilli loses its germinative properties and does not mature.

Infection through the Placenta.—The passage of tubercle bacilli through the intact placental tissue is still a disputed question. CORNET [3] considers the normal placenta as an impenetrable filter to corpuscular elements and bacteria, but believes that infectious diseases, accompanied by high fever, may produce epithelial defects which render the passage of the bacteria into the fœtal organism possible. The same author also makes the statement, that in case of a tuberculous mother, such a passage is apparently only possible, if a tuberculous focus is located in the placenta itself. This restriction does not seem logical because if the possibility of the discontinuity of the placental lining is to be accepted, the recent discovery of tubercle bacilli in the circulating blood of tuberculous patients would make it possible for them to pass without the presence of any actual lesion.

The placental lining undoubtedly is one of the most impenetrable structures of the human organism. It does not permit the passage of any of the corpuscular elements of the blood. The virus of smallpox may pass, as proven by the fact that children have been born with signs of the disease. But an analogy from this cannot be drawn as to tuberculous infection. The causative agent of the former is unknown, while the latter disease is caused by quite an appreciable organism.

Congenital Infection Rare.—The comparatively few cases of authentic congenital infection on record, have nearly all been associated with tuberculous disease of the placenta. This is, without a doubt, the most common method of parental infection and does not require a hypothetical supposition of discontinuity between the individual cells of the placental lining.

A tuberculous disease of the placenta may cause ulceration of the vessels with subsequent dispersal of the bacilli in the fœtal organism, or tubercles in the placenta may be broken up at birth, and the particles thus enter the portal vessels.

HARBITZ [4] considers infection before birth extremely rare and believes that if a child of one to three months has lived even for a short time in a tuberculous environment, no conclusion can be drawn as to whether the infection occurred before or after birth.

The rarity of congenital transmission of tuberculosis is seen by the fact that the extended researches in the literature by such men as HARBITZ and CORNET resulted only in the finding of 20 to 30 authenticated cases. HARBITZ [5] collected 20, CORNET [6] 26, and SCHLUETER [7] 20 cases respectively. The rarity of the condition is illustrated by MEDIN's [8] series of 7,630 autopsies of infants under one year with 623 cases of tuberculosis among which only one would lead to suspicion of being of congenital origin.

v. Baumgarten's Views not Supported.—v. Baumgarten is one of the few men who places marked importance on the congenital transmission of this disease; he bases his theory on the experiments of FRIEDMAN [9] who found in animals bacilli mixed with the sperm, which was thus transferred to the foetus and later into the different organs, while the mother remained free from tuberculosis. The same observer also has found an infected ovum within the ovary from a case of maternal tuberculosis.

But to base such a far-reaching theory upon the experiments of a single observer seems rather irrational. Many other men have failed to confirm them. But v. Baumgarten also lays stress on placental transmission and believes that it is in the early stages of placental disease before the lesions are easily recognized that transmission of the bacillus takes place. This author then explains the further course of the disease by a theory of latency and insusceptibility of the infant tissues to the formation of the tubercle, owing to their great activity in growth.

But the acute course of infant tuberculosis in general speaks against this supposition, also the very rare occurrence of a positive tuberculin test in newborn children. The earliest ever recorded is that of ZARFL,[10] who reported a positive v. Pirquet test in a 17 days' old child.

BRONCHOGENOUS INFECTION

The great frequency of involvement of the Bronchial Glands speaks for the importance of the aërogenous infection. CAMBY in a series of 569 cases of tuberculosis found the bronchial glands involved in all; HAMBURGER and LENKE found the same condition in 110 cases, HAUSHALTER and FRUHINSHOLZ in 74 out of 78 infants dying of acute tuberculosis, or tuberculous meningitis.[11] Modern investigations seem to prove that in the great majority of cases of bronchial gland tuberculosis, the primary lesion is to be found in the lung. HEDREN [12] in his series of 690 autopsies on children found 199 cases of tuberculosis, of these 47 were infants under one year, and 152 were over one year. The 47 infants had the bronchial glands involved in 100%, and the lungs in 98% of the cases; the older children had the bronchial glands involved in 93.4% and the lungs in 91.4%. HEDREN places great importance upon the fact that in nearly all of his cases the step-like progress from the portal of entry could be established and remarks that the few exceptions probably were only apparent. GHON [13] in his series of 184 autopsies on tuberculous children showed, by very scrupulous examination of the lungs, that the bronchial gland lesions were accompanied by older pulmonary lesions. PARROTT [14] tried to prove that there does not exist any "tracheo-bronchial" adenopathy which is not of pulmonary origin: "Every time a bronchial gland is the seat of a tuberculous lesion, there is a tuberculous lesion in the lung." In MEDIN's series of 623 autopsies of tuberculous infants under one year, 98% showed primary involvement of lungs and bronchial glands.

From these facts it would seem that the aërogenous route is mostly concerned in production of bronchial gland tuberculosis although the arguments of v. BEHRING and CALMETTE, and others are not to be lightly thrown away.

Bronchial Gland Infection May be Primary.—Although GHON's and HEDREN's findings seem to indicate that a pulmonary lesion is always present in case of hilus tuberculosis, many investigators believe that the tubercle bacilli are able to penetrate the pulmonary epithelial lining without producing any change and thus primarily attack the bronchial glands where they are retained.

The bacilli enter with the inspired air, either in the form of dust or droplets and lodge on the mucous membrane of the bronchioles or pulmonary alveoli. A local process may set up with subsequent, secondary involvement of the bronchial glands, or the bacilli may pass the epithelial lining, enter the lymph-stream and be propelled to the pulmonary or broncho-pulmonary glands. WOLLSTEIN and BARTLETT [15] hold this latter theory far more tenable; in their series of 178 cases of tuberculosis, 14 existed without any pulmonary lesion, but with involvement of the bronchial glands. HEDREN and GHON consider the primary lesion in the lung overlooked in these cases. But whatever the case may be, the bronchial glands certainly have been shown to be the true center of infantile tuberculosis, from which the disease may spread in various ways.

ENTEROGENOUS MODE OF INFECTION

Mechanism of Intestinal Absorption.—The intestinal or alimentary infection undoubtedly plays an important part in children, especially in infants. This is proven by the great number of primary infections of the mesenteric glands, which have been demonstrated by numerous investigators. Without accepting the radical views of v. BEHRING and CALMETTE who contend that the majority of the cases of tuberculosis are caused by enterogenous infection, we will consider the mechanism of intestinal absorption of tubercle bacilli as put forth by CALMETTE.[16] In the lower animals, which possess a digestive sac, the cells of the endoderm send out toward the interior of the cavity pseudopods resembling those of the amœba and which engulf solid particles of food. The enormous absorbing surface of the digestive canal in higher animals is lined nearly throughout with similar cells having the same properties. They line the small and large intestines. We know that during the process of digestion, divers protein substances, fatty acids and glycerin, solid particles and bacteria are constantly entering the intestinal villi. This process is realized by the intervention of migratory cells, which penetrate the cylindrical cells of the intestinal epithelium. This process is especially intense in Peyers patches. When the microörganism carried by the leucocyte, has penetrated into a lacteal vessel, it follows the current of lymph towards the nearest lymph-gland, the mesenteric. In the glands the lymph-current is markedly slowed down, due to their peculiar anatomy. If the bacilli are numerous and virulent, or if they have had time to multiply, a typical glandular tuberculosis is produced.

Glands Act as Filters.—In the young, the glands act as nearly perfect filters, and thus retain the germs, especially in case of massive infection. A tuberculous lesion is soon produced which becomes caseous and distributes the microörganisms in the different lymphatics and blood-stream.

But if the infecting bacilli were less numerous or less virulent, the leucocytes which had engulfed them would remain uninjured, conserve their mobility and continue their migration in the lymphatic or blood-vascular network of the different organs until they lose their vitality. In older animals the lymph-glands are of looser texture, and often more permeable than in the young; the bacilli always engulfed by the leucocytes are carried with the lymph of the thoracic duct into the blood of the right heart and distributed in the pulmonary capillaries. The leucocytes having lost more or less of their vitality, are caught acting as emboli. The tubercle bacilli contained in these leucocytes, produce the typical changes.

The Intestinal Mucosa is Permeable.—Experiments, demonstrating the passage of tubercle bacilli through the healthy intestinal mucous membrane, have been performed by various investigators. CHAVEAU and DOBROKLOWSKI [17] were amongst the first to insist upon the ease with which the tuberculous virus traversed the healthy epithelial lining without causing any apparent lesion. That bacteria of various kinds passed the intestinal mucous membrane, especially during digestion of fatty material, was proven by DESOURBY and PORCHER [17] who recovered the bacteria in the chyle and blood several hours later.

Infection by Direct Inoculation.—RAVENEL, V. BEHRING and ROEMER, BISANTI and PANISSET, FICKER, OBERWORTH and L. RABINOWITSCH [17] have found that following an infectious meal not only the lymph but also the blood frequently contained the tubercle bacilli. SCHLOSSMAN, ENGEL, ORTH and RABINO-

WITSCH [17] have demonstrated after animals have been infected by direct inoculation into the stomach, through an abdominal incision, that the lungs of these animals six hours after inoculation contained virus capable of infecting other animals.

L. Findley's Experiment.—Findley [18] performed a series of experiments to ascertain what part the intestines play as a portal of entry for the tubercle bacillus. He suspended cultures of bovine and human bacilli in oil, enclosed them in gelatine capsules which he introduced through a stomach tube into the stomachs of healthy rabbits and rabbits which had recently suffered from intestinal catarrh. Findley draws the following conclusions from his experiments:

Healthy rabbits can be infected by ingestion of large amounts of bovine tubercle bacilli.

The bacilli can pass through apparently intact intestinal mucous membrane and reach the mesenteric glands within a period of six days.

When infection occurs the intestine is invariably the seat of the lesions and thus tuberculosis of any organ other than the intestine is always a secondary infection when the bacilli have entered by the intestinal route.

Catarrh of the intestines does not favor the passage of tubercle bacilli through the wall, but allows of a more constant and widespread infection and in this way facilitates dissemination. Healthy rabbits apparently cannot be infected by the ingestion of large amounts of the human tubercle bacilli. Rabbits just recovered from intestinal catarrh develop tuberculosis after the ingestion of human tubercle bacilli. With the human organism, a local lesion, though always present, may be slight in comparison with the diseased foci in the mesenteric glands.

Walsham's Views.—WALSHAM [19] in his work on the channels of infection in tuberculosis comes to the conclusion that the mesenteric glands may be found to be tuberculous without there being any discoverable lesion in the intestine, and believes that the explanation must be accepted, that the bacilli are carried by the leucocytes, along the lymph-channels to the heart and lung.

Objections to the Intestinal Routes of Infection.—v. BEHR-

ING's and CALMETTE's contention that the great majority of cases of tuberculosis are spread by the intestinal mode of infection is hotly contested by the majority of investigators.

v. PIRQUET [20] believes that the enterogenous infection has been much overestimated. He considers intestinal tuberculous invasion in infants very common but, as a rule, secondary and due to the deglutition of tuberculous mucus, which comes from the lungs.

Intestinal Tract not Susceptible to Infection.—CORNET [21] is of the opinion that the intestinal tract, of all organs of the body, is the least accessible to tuberculous infection, not on account of any insusceptibility of its mucous membrane, but rather on account of the quick passage of the infected material which does not allow the bacilli to get a firm hold, or to settle, and also on account of the mixing with the intestinal contents.

COBBET [22] does not believe that the experiments of VANSTEEN-BERCHE and GRYSEZ, who found anthracosis of the lungs after feeding guinea-pigs india ink and carbon, were conclusive. He considers the anthracosis as a natural condition of the city-bred pigs. COBBET failed to verify the experiments on country-bred guinea-pigs.

One of the most forcible objections against the importance of intestinal infection is that brought forth by CHAUSSÉ, FLÜGGE and FINDEL.[23] The latter showed that the number of bacilli required to produce infection of the alimentary tract was very much larger than that to cause infection by inhalation. After several experiments he concluded that the minimum fatal dose in ingestion is about 6 times greater than the minimum fatal dose in inhalation. CALMETTE does not believe that this objection is tenable, because nothing proves that one virulent bacillus absorbed in the intestine is sufficient to produce a tuberculous lesion.

Frequency of Intestinal Infection.—The reports on frequency of primary intestinal infection vary markedly in different countries. European investigators in general find a comparatively low frequency. ALBRECHT in examining 1,080 cases found only seven primary intestinal infections; GHON [24] examining 180 odd cases found three; v. HAUSEMANN [25] twenty-five in 10,000 autopsies; HUNTER thirteen cases amongst 5,124; BIEDERT [25] sixteen amongst 3,104 children. MEDIN in his series of 623 tuberculous infants under one year, found primary intestinal tuberculosis in two per cent of the cases and hence considers it of little importance in infants. HEDREN [26] found eleven cases of undisputable deglutition tuberculosis amongst 199 tuberculous children and concludes that although the condition is comparatively rare, its importance should not be overlooked. BOVAIRD [27] of New York refers to 1,161 post-mortem examinations of tuberculous children among which he found 2.05% suffering from primary intestinal tuberculosis.

GAFFNEY and ROTHE [28] examined 400 cases by inoculating parts of bronchial and mesenteric glands into guinea-pigs. They found 78 positive cases—19.5%. In 42 cases both groups were involved—54%, in 14 cases the mesenteric glands only were involved—18%, while the bronchial glands only were involved in 22 cases—28%. WOLLSTEIN and BARTLETT [29] of New York in their series of 1,320 autopsies with 178 cases of tuberculosis found primary intestinal lesions in 9.5%. W. H. PARK [30] in his collected series of 1,500 cases found abdominal tuberculosis or generalized tuberculosis of alimentary origin in 107 cases—7.13%. COUNCILMAN of Boston found 37% primary intestinal lesions. HELLER of Kiel 37.8%, BEITZKE 16—20%, and PRICE-JONES 25%.[31]

Bovine Bacilli, Evidence of Primary Alimentary Infection.— One of the best criterions for primary infection of the alimentary tract is the actual presence of bovine infection. MITCHELL [32] in eight cases of abdominal tuberculosis in children under twelve years of age, found the bovine type of tubercle bacillus seven times and the human type once; all these children had been fed on raw cow's milk. WOODHEAD [33] believes that a considerable proportion of cases of tuberculosis of the alimentary canal and of the adjacent lymph-glands is the result of bovine infection. Even CORNET admits that small as the danger is in individual cases, the multiplicity of opportunities gives it considerable importance for children.

Secondary infection of the alimentary tract is much more common than the primary. It is then due to swallowing tuberculous mucus which comes from the lungs. It occurs especially in the later stages of the disease and results often in marked involvement of the intestinal wall with subsequent changes in the mesenteric glands.

INFECTION OF THE EXTERNAL LYMPH-GLANDS

Of the external lymph-glands the cervical are the ones most often affected with tuberculosis; the following tables by BALMANN and WOHLGEMUTH [34] give us a conception of the relative frequency of the involvement of the different glands:

	Balmann	Wohlgemuth
Neck and Occipital Glands	81 %	93 %
Axillary "	6 %	2.78%
Inguinal "	7 %	0.93%
Ulner "	5 %	0.23%
Popliteal "	0.7%	0.23%
In front and behind ear	– %	2.9 %

Cervical Glands.—The greater preponderance of cervical gland involvement is undoubtedly due to greater opportunities for infection. Their area of drainage is most commonly exposed, the upper respiratory and digestive passages receiving the brunt of the attack, whether the infection is conveyed by the aërogenous route, or by food or drink.

Portals of Entry. Palatine Tonsils.—The tonsils and the adjacent area are drained by the superior deep cervical glands, and according to WOOD, especially by the ones lying under the anterior border of the Sterno-cleido-mastoid muscle, just behind the angle of the mandible. These glands form part of the mesial group of the superior deep cervical glands, which group is usually the one most commonly affected. MOST considers infection of the palatine tonsil and its vicinity, of the greatest etiological importance.

Waldeyer's Ring, The First Line of Defense.—The situation of the tonsil is such that any bacilli entering the mouth and being swallowed, pass over its surface and may gain entrance to the crypts. The tonsillar ring of WALDEYER, as a whole, undoubtedly plays an important rôle as a first line of defense against infection, and whatever it cannot handle is propelled along the lymph-stream to the next line, the lymph-glands, where they produce the characteristic changes.

Sclerosed Tonsils a Menace.—The opinion that only the hypertrophied tonsil can be the source of infection seems scarcely reasonable, in view of the fact that repeated inflammatory attacks of the tonsils often leave them sclerosed and atrophic and hence less able to deal with microörganisms than when they are of normal size.[35]   The small sclerosed tonsil may increase the facility of infection, because of its crypts having wider openings on the buccal surface than normal; also because of atrophy of the lymphatic tissue.

Frequency of Tonsillar Tuberculosis.—Numerous investigations have been made with regard to tuberculosis of the tonsil. Various authors have collected thousands of cases, the average findings running quite parallel. In cases where no tuberculous symptoms are present, examination of the tonsils reveals the presence of tuberculosis in from 4 to 6%.

LOCKHARD [36] collected 1,988 cases of pharyngeal and faucial tonsillar enlargements and found tuberculosis in 5.9%. WOOD [37] collected 1,671 cases from the literature with tuberculosis in 5.2%. GÖRDELER [38] reported 47 cases with 12.75% of tuberculosis.   PYBUS [39] collected 751 cases with 6.7% positive. STREET [40] examined 100 pairs of tonsils removed from supposedly non-tuberculous patients; 10% of these tonsils showed tuberculous processes in different stages of development.

Association Between Diseased Tonsils and Cervical Glands.— Examination of the tonsils associated with enlarged cervical glands reveals a higher frequency of tuberculosis. NICOLL [41] examined 500 cases of chronic enlargement of the cervical lymph-glands in children and a great number of hyperplastic tonsils which showed signs of simple inflammation and found tuberculosis in 80%. He believes that in 80% of the enlarged lymph-glands the cause for the tuberculous involvement is to be found in the hyperplasia of the tonsils. LOCKHARD estimates it at 90%, GARDINER and PYBUS 80%. But these estimations seem rather high. Actual findings are much less. GARDINER [42] in examining tonsils associated with cervical adenitis found tuberculosis in 4 out of 30 cases. CARMICHAEL [43] 7 out of 50 cases, KINGS-FORD [44] 7 out of 17, MITCHELL [44] 24 out of 73, and HURD and WRIGHT [44] 9 out of 12 cases, which gives us an average of 28.17%.

In a recent article MITCHELL again shows that primary tuberculosis of the faucial tonsils is by no means so rare as is generally supposed and according to the same author the importance of recognizing it as a primary focus cannot be too strongly insisted upon. In 106 cases of tuberculous cervical glands, the tonsils were found to be tuberculous in 38%. In this series 51 cases were found to have small and submerged tonsils, 27 hypertrophied and 28 tonsils of medium size. In 100 cases of hypertrophied tonsils with barely palpable cervical glands 9% were found to be tuberculous.

CORNET [44] does not believe that we are justified in attaching any great importance to the tonsils as a portal of entrance in tuberculosis of the cervical glands, to say nothing of making them almost entirely answerable for their causation; other authors, on the other hand, notably AUFRECHT and GROBER [45] consider the tonsil to be one of the most frequent points of entry of tuberculosis, and that tuberculosis of the lungs arises from them.

The feeding experience of GRIFFITH [46] include a total of 92 animals and give us undoubtedly a true conception of the conditions at hand.

TABULATED ACCOUNT OF GRIFFITH'S EXPERIMENTS

Species of Animals	Number fed with the material	Number tonsils tbc	Number neck glands tbc	Number Int. tbc	Mesent. and colic gl. tbc
Chimpanzees	7	1	4	7	7
Rhesus monks	7	1	4	7	7
Baboons	14	9	11	13	13
Calves	21	3	5	16	20
Goats	9	1	5	2	8
Pigs	34	8	21	10	32
TOTAL	92	23	50	55	87

The tonsils in this series then show an involvement of 25%, while the neck glands are involved in 54.3%. The conclusions would then not seem very far from the truth, that in cases of cervical tuberculous adenitis, the tonsils are responsible for the condition in about 50% of the cases.

Secondary tuberculosis of the tonsils is more common than the primary. It may be the result of infection from germ-laden sputum, occurring then in the later stages of pulmonary tuberculosis, or it may appear in the course of miliary tuberculosis, then being due to infection through the blood-stream. In either case it may be accompanied by involvement of the cervical glands. PYBUS [47] collected 115 cases (Strassman, Kruckmann, Walsham and Friedman) in which examination of the tonsils had been made in those dying from tuberculosis and found 70 positive cases or 60.8%; in those who died, 55 cases, the tonsils were tuberculous in 96.4%.

Pharyngeal Tonsil.—The Pharyngeal tonsil or the tonsil of Luschke, is located in the vault of the nasopharynx. Hypertrophy of this mass of lymphoid tissue is commonly known as adenoids. This condition, probably due to repeated irritations from the inspired air, forms a favorable spot for the deposit of various bacteria contained in the air. The air current, changing its direction in the vault of the pharynx, is thrown directly on to the tonsils. This uneven structure, with its many crypts, is especially suitable for retention of bacteria and is undoubtedly responsible for a certain number of cases of cervical adenitis.

Tuberculous infection of the pharyngeal tonsils is more complicated than that of the palatine tonsils. Primary infection may occur through the inspired air, but infection through food is impossible, hence hardly any opportunity for bovine infection. Secondary infection by means of sputum is very difficult, due to closure of the posterior nares during attacks of coughing; but, of course, infection can take place through the expired air.

The actual presence of tuberculosis in the pharyngeal tonsils is estimated differently by various authors. Some go so far as to consider this tonsil the most important and most common portal of entry for the tubercle bacilli, notably BECKMANN. BLUMENFIELD [48] does not take this extreme view, but believes that the adenoid growths play a definite rôle in producing tuberculous adenitis both in the cervical and bronchial regions.

Examinations of the adenoids reduce the frequency to quite an extent. LACHMANN [49] collected 2,065 cases with histological examinations and inoculation experiments and found tuberculosis 89 times, or 4.3%. SIMON [50] collected 1,361 cases with 67 positive, i. e., about 5%. Hence the proportion is quite comparable with tuberculous involvement of the faucial tonsils.

Mucous Membrane of Nose, Mouth and Pharynx.—According to CORNET and MOST the mucous membrane of the nose does not form a negligible portal of entry for the tubercle bacillus. It is, without question, one of the most exposed mucous membranes in the human body. The germ-laden inspired air is constantly passing over it and catarrhal conditions of the nose are common enough to render it more or less an easy prey for the penetration of the tubercle bacilli.

Calmette's Views.—But, as CALMETTE [51] remarks, the nasal mucous membrane does not permit the penetration of tubercle bacilli as easily as one would believe, in spite of the rich network of lymphatics and veins, in spite of the enormous quantities of dust of all sorts, which accumulate with each inspiration. The reason is, according to the same author, that these foreign particles exercise a positive chemotaxis upon the leucocytes; these leave the capillaries to engulf them, but before they reach them they are immobilized and captured on the surface of the mucous membrane, due to the sticky mucus produced by the glands. Deprived of their motion the leucocytes cannot again enter the circulation but are expelled with the mucus. Proof of this is that tubercle bacilli are often found in the nasal cavities of perfectly sound individuals and that primary infection of the nasal mucosa is very rare.

Lockard's Views.—LOCKARD [52] supposes that since infection is rarest at the point naturally most exposed to infection, one must assume for the nasal mucous membrane, or its secretions, some strong inherent power of defense. He enumerates the following properties of the nasal mucosa and its secretions as having an important bearing upon the rarity of nasal infection.

The peculiar character of the nasal secretion which renders it antagonistic to the life or growth of morbific germs. The extreme sensitiveness and reflex irritability of the nasal mucous membrane, whereby the inhalation of any irritant provokes almost instantaneous congestion, swelling of the erectile tissues and increased flow of the watery secretions, with probable expulsion of the foreign elements.

The increased flow of secretions and the action of the cilia, plus the almost constant presence of a film of mucus, renders the nasal mucous membrane almost a negligible factor as a portal of entry for tuberculous infection.

The mucous membrane of the mouth and pharynx with the exception of the tonsillar region, oppose the infection in the same manner as the nasal mucous membrane. Tuberculous lesions of this area are quite rare; the tongue may sometimes be affected, also the gums; the pharynx proper is very rarely the seat of primary infection.[53] But the possibility of bacillary penetration is not to be entirely overlooked.

Cornet's Experiments.—CORNET believes that the rôle played by this part of the mucous membrane is quite important in production of cervical adenitis. In his experiments on animals, he produced tuberculosis of the cervical glands by rubbing the gums, back of the pharynx and the tongue, with tuberculous material without any changes whatever occurring at the point of inoculations. JOUSSET [54] is of the opinion that the chief portal of entry for the tubercle bacilli is the upper parts of the digestive and respiratory tracts, namely, the mucous membrane of the nose, throat and tonsils. MEDIN [55] believes that the mucous membrane of the nose and pharynx plays a very insignificant rôle as portal of entry in infants.

The Teeth.—The mouth has long been known to be the most septic of all cavities in the human body, still it is only lately that oral sepsis has begun to receive the attention that it deserves. The loose carious teeth in children are undoubtedly the greatest danger; with their open pulp channels and ulcerating sockets, they are portals for the entrance of pathogenic bacteria of every description.

That the teeth in children have been, up to the present time, the most neglected members of the body by both the physician and the dentist, there can be no question. I believe that in the near future it will be demonstrated that the present methods of treatment of diseased deciduous teeth is far from perfect. With the exception of the tonsils, it is the teeth and their immediate root-coverings that, without question, furnish the most important portals of entry for infection. BLAIR [56] describes three distinct routes:

1—Open pulp canal
2—Diseased peridental membrane
3—Injuries to surrounding tissues by the
   sharp edges of carious crowns and roots.

Relation between Carious Teeth and Cervical Adenitis.—The relation between carious teeth and tuberculous cervical glands has repeatedly been proven. STARCK [57] examined 113 children with cervical adenitis, and proved that 41% of the examined cases were due to carious teeth, by demonstrating the presence of the same organism in the gland, teeth and the connecting lymphatic vessels in some cases, or by showing the local dependence of the glandular swelling upon the situation of the carious tooth; caries of the posterior molars were associated with swellings of the posterior submaxillary glands—the canine teeth with those of the anterior gland. PEDLEY [58] examined 3,145 children and found carious teeth present in 77.5% of the cases, associated with more or less pronounced cervical lymphadenitis.

Odenthal's Findings.—ODENTHAL [59] examined 978 children, 429 of which had progressive caries of the teeth; all of these, except four, had cervical lymphadenitis. In 237 cases the teeth were badly broken down and the glandular swellings more pronounced. In 359 cases no cause of the enlarged glands could be assigned except carious teeth. In 131 cases caries were found on one side only, and the enlarged glands on the same side. KÖRNER [60] examined 1,645 children and demonstrated the correspondence of the glandular enlargement with the affected tooth both as to position and degree of infection.

Starck's Case.—Absolute proofs are not lacking to show the dependence in some cases of tuberculous cervical adenitis, upon carious teeth. Take for instance a case reported by STARCK [61]— an 18-year-old boy suddenly developed toothache on the left side; after a certain period of time a swelling beneath the left jaw developed and gradually increased in size; the gland was proven to be tuberculous and tubercle bacilli were found in the carious tooth. ENLER [62] had one case in which the track from the tooth to the tuberculous granuloma could be traced by the microscope.

Tubercle Bacilli Found in Carious Teeth.—Tubercle bacilli have, a number of times, been found in carious teeth. COOK [63] examined 220 mouths—saliva, decayed teeth and root-pulps, and found tubercle bacilli in eleven cases, in some associated with pulmonary tuberculosis, or cervical lymphadenitis—in some associated with no demonstrable tuberculosis anywhere.

Moorehead's Findings.—MOOREHEAD [64] has reported several cases of cervical lymphadenitis with carious teeth and the actual findings of tubercle bacilli in the decayed root-pulps. MOELLER [65] lays stress on the importance of carious teeth and ulcers of unclean mouths as portals of entry. He examined 53 healthy children and found carious teeth in 26 cases, and foul conditions of the mouth in 41 cases. No tubercle bacilli were found in the teeth, but six times in the sordes, while pseudotubercle bacilli were found nine times in the teeth and eighteen times in the sordes. Amongst 194 children with diseased lungs he found 153 cases of carious teeth and 182 cases of ulcerations of the mouth. Tubercle bacilli were found 14 times in the teeth and 35 times in the ulcerations, while pseudotubercle bacilli were found 23 and 42 times respectively.

Wright's Views.—A point brought out by WRIGHT [66] that undoubtedly has an important bearing on this question is the presence of hemolytic streptococci so often causing small abscesses around the root ends. These germs lower the vitality of the tissues and through their hemolytic action on the blood, and adjacent structures render a pathway for the invasion of tubercle bacilli. These statements certainly go to show that carious teeth play a more or less important rôle in the production of tuberculous cervical adenitis; the exposed pulp furnishes an open avenue for infection, no covering mucous membrane being present to impede its progress. The presence of lymphatics has been definitely proven by SCHWEIZER and hence an open road exists to the submaxillary glands which are intimately connected with the deep cervical.

Eye, Ear and Skin.—Experiments on animals have proven [67] (Calmette, Cornet) that tubercle bacilli may pass the conjunctival mucous membrane without producing any changes at the place of entry, but soon being followed by the development of a typical adenitis. In man the conjunctiva is drained by the parotid and submaxillary lymph-glands, the second station being the superficial and deep cervical glands. This mode of infection hardly plays an important rôle in the production of tuberculous cervical adenitis. Chances for infection are common enough by means of dirty fingers, handkerchiefs, etc., but the protecting influence of the lacrimal secretion and the nearly perfect drainage provided by the flow of tears undoubtedly forms a barrier which is hard to overcome by such a slowly progressing affair as a tuberculous infection.

Middle Ear and Mastoid.—Primary tuberculosis of the middle ear occurs most readily in children, and according to BANDELIER and ROEPKE [68] is limited to those cases in which chronic middle ear suppurations afford a favorable ground for infection, which may occur either from outside through a perforation in the membrane, or through the eustachian tube. FORDYCE and CARMICHAEL [69] call particular attention to the danger of aspiration up the eustachian tube during the act of sucking, hence giving another pathway for bovine infection in artificially fed babies.

Primary tuberculosis of the mastoid is quite frequent in children, 15% of all cases of inflammatory mastoid disease being tuberculous.[70]

The lymph-glands involved in these cases are the auricular and retro-pharyngeal, from which the process travels to the deep cervical.

Skin of the Face.—Of all the organs of the human body the skin is the one which offers the least favorable conditions for the penetration of the tubercle bacilli. In spite of the frequent contact with infected material, tuberculosis of the skin is quite rare. Experimentally the tuberculous infection can be made to traverse the skin, but only after marked rubbing whereby some slight superficial erosion has been produced. The skin of the face is often the seat of small lesions, such as cracks, fissures, eczematous patches. Through these infections may take place.

Scheltema's Case.—SCHELTEMA [71] reports the case of an eight weeks' old child who had a tuberculous lesion of the forehead and involvement of the regional lymph-glands. This infant had had a wound on the forehead and had been taken care of by a tuberculous father. The sequence of events is obvious. CHANCELLOR [72] reports two cases: A two months' old baby was bitten on the cheek by a tuberculous nurse, an ulcer developed with subsequent swelling of the maxillary and cervical lymph-glands. A one-year old boy was wounded on the neck and infected by an uncle who had positive sputum; ulceration with subsequent cervical adenitis followed. Cases are on record where infection has taken place through the wound caused by piercing the ear-lobe for earrings.

The Scalp, and Pediculosis.—The scalp may sometimes furnish the atrium for tuberculous infection with subsequent involvement of the occipital and deep cervical glands. Pediculosis undoubtedly plays some rôle in these cases, although the condition is, as a rule, associated with eczematous lesions of the scalp.

Infection of the Pre-laryngeal Glands.—The Pre-laryngeal gland, or glands, located in front of the crico-thyroid membrane, is often involved in cases of endo-laryngeal tuberculosis and may cause involvement of the deep cervical glands, due to the connection existing between the two groups.

Infection of the Axillary Glands.—The Axillary glands drain the skin of the upper part of the thoracic wall, the upper abdominal region and the upper extremities. They are also connected with the lateral group of the inferior deep cervical glands. The avenues of infection of this group of glands, are then apparent. The infection through the upper extremity is relatively rare.

Jousset [73] reports how he infected himself with virulent bovine bacilli through a wound in the finger; a few days later a tuberculous nodule appeared with swelling of the axillary lymph-glands. It occurs generally in the course of tuberculosis of the bones of the hand and arms.

Infection of the Mammary Glands.—Tuberculous infection of the mammary gland is, as a rule, according to Most,[74] due to tuberculosis of a rib with subsequent infection of the skin. Because connection exists between the lateral group of the supra-clavicular or inferior deep cervical glands and the axillary glands, infection of the latter may sometimes be the result of spreading of the disease from the former.

Infection of the Inguinal Glands.—Tuberculosis of the genital organs is associated with inguinal adenitis. The female genetalia are more commonly affected than the male. In infants infection may take place during the process of cleansing, and later by introduction of various foreign bodies. In the male, the most common mode, although rare, is through the ritual circumcision. Holt [75] collected 41 cases from the literature in which the operation had been performed in the usual manner, the blood being sucked by the operator. In nearly all of these cases the respective families were free from tuberculosis, while the operator, on the other hand, was tuberculous. Ulceration of the operating wound was the result, with subsequent swelling of the inguinal glands.

Tuberculosis of the anal mucous membrane is usually a secondary affair, although primary cases are on record; the inguinal glands draining this area are subsequently involved.

Rôle of the Lymph-Glands in Tuberculous Infection in Children.—It is evident that the lymph-glands play a very important part in the struggle of the organism against infection with tuberculosis, especially in children, who are particularly liable to infection. By reason of their location near the periphery of the body and in positions exposed to infection, they may be said to constitute a second line of defense against the infection.

They Act as Filters.—Because of their anatomical structure they are well adapted to act as protective organs and filters to the lymph-stream, being composed of masses of lymphoid cells encapsulated with fibrous tissue and possessed of small portals of exit. In children the glands are better fitted to combat infection than in adults because of the greater abundance of lymphoid cells and the lesser amount of fibrous tissue. The lymph-glands form, on account of their capsules, organs which are entirely enclosed except for the afferent and efferent vessels. Toxins produced by retained bacteria will therefore not diffuse themselves so readily into surrounding tissues. The concentration of the toxins hinders the growth of the bacteria and causes a reaction of the tissue, coagulation necrosis resulting, which, together with stasis and thrombosis of the lymph and blood-vessels, aids in the prevention of further dispersal of the bacteria.

The lymph-glands often sacrifice their existence for the protection of the organism. The fact that the lymph-glands advance the infection less than the other organs cannot be denied. In infancy the lymphatic system is the part which possesses relatively the greatest power of resistance, but in spite of this, it is not capable of withstanding the assault of the tubercle bacillus and there is a marked tendency to rapid and general dissemination and healing rarely occurs. The reaction is insufficient and the glands fail to arrest the bacilli, which spread through the lymphatic system, attack other tissues and cause a fatal termination. Miliary tuberculosis and tuberculous meningitis are comparatively frequent and evidence of this tendency to dissemination.

Glandular tuberculosis in adults is of less importance, but the rôle it plays in childhood is very great and it is now generally believed that the tuberculosis of the adult is a later stage of the glandular infection in childhood.

In most cases of primary infection of older children, the tubercle bacilli do not penetrate beyond the regional lymph-glands. With caseation and the production of allergy the infection is overcome completely or temporarily.

MORBID ANATOMY

Formation of the Tubercle.—When the tubercle attacks any organ or tissue the reaction is twofold. One constitutes the response of the organism to the invading bacilli and consists of productive and protective changes; the other is degenerative in character and is the result of the destructive action of the infective agent.

The commonest product of the tubercle bacillus is the tubercle. It represents a new growth in the affected tissue and consists, at least during the initial stages, of derivatives of fixed tissue cells. The condition is analogous to simple inflammation in which exudative and cellular processes are the result of the action of an irritant.

Proliferative processes play the most important rôle. The first result of the invasion of the tissue is a mitosis of connective tissue and endothelial cells, resulting in the formation of epithelioid cells. They are so called because they form a dense mass and are connected like epithelial cells. Their mutual arrangement is their distinguishing feature, and they are comparable to the fibroclasts of simple inflammation. The blood-vessels in the immediate neighborhood are almost always occluded by compression or by the ingrowth of tubercle into their wall.

Giant Cell Formation.—The epithelioid cells may be converted into giant cells. Their formation may in general be regarded as the expression of a diminished vital activity. Two types may be considered, according to the method of their formation.[76]

First, the proliferation giant cells in which rapid nuclear division, often amitotic, occurs without division of the cell body; second, the conglutination giant cell formed by the fusion of two or more epithelioid cells. When the tubercle has grown to be just visible to the naked eye other elements gather at the periphery. Small round cells accumulate at first in or around the peripheral zone, and contribute to the enlargement of the nodule; later they invade its central portions. They are small round cells with deeply staining nuclei and small proto-plasmic bodies and are derived from the blood-vessels. During late stages polymorphous nuclear leucocytes also appear in addition to the mononuclear forms. They collect in large numbers at the periphery. In addition to the cellular elements a variable quantity of fibrin is deposited in the central and peripheral parts of the tubercle.

The tubercle has a delicate fibrillar reticulum partly derived from the fibrous ground substance of the tissue and in part from newly formed fibers. No new blood-vessels are formed in the structure and the ones involved are occluded and destroyed by pressure of the epithelioid cells.

Degenerative changes soon set in, the cause for which is to be sought in the toxic products produced by the infective agent and in the avascular condition of the tubercle. These changes begin in the centre of the tuberculous nodule and progress in concentric lines toward its periphery. The giant and epithelioid cells are first to undergo destruction and the leucocytic elements soon follow. The degenerative changes result in caseation necrosis in which the protoplasm fails to stain and shows granular and fatty degeneration. The nuclei become fragmented and stain lightly or not at all, and the final result is a dry, firm, bloodless mass. In the end the necrosis involves the fibrous network and the trabeculæ of fibrin.

Foci Undergo Caseation.—Foci which have undergone complete caseation frequently become the seat of secondary deposits of calcareous salts. In small nodules almost complete absorption may result. The tubercle may become encapsulated by fibrous changes. The epithelioid cells are genetically connective tissue cells and they may undergo transformation, lengthen and develop fibroblasts and connective tissue, converting the tubercle into a purely fibrous structure. A certain amount of secondary connective tissue formation occurs in the surrounding tissue.

Tuberculosis of the lymphatic glands is not always associated with the typical tubercle formation. The earliest change is often simple hyperplasia with consequent swelling. In certain cases the only change may be one of hyperplasia characterized by the transformation of the normal gland tissue into large celled tissue, having none of the characteristics of the original structure and consisting partly of rounded and polygonal cells and partly of spindle cells. Such glands remain discrete and may resemble those of Hodgkin's disease. There is little tendency to caseation except in the late stages. BARTEL [77] was able to demonstrate in the lymph-glands of animals, in addition to manifest tuberculosis in the specific tuberculous changes, a stage of lymphoid tuberculosis in which the glands showed mainly lymphatic hyperplasia or were but little changed. The picture suggests infection of low virulence.

Glandular Chains Involved.—Any of the lymph-glands of the body may be involved but the cervical, tracheo-bronchial and mesenteric·glands are most often affected, by reason of their draining areas of the mucous membranes of the body which are the most common portals of entry of the tubercle bacillus. The glandular infection is usually lymphogenous, rarely hematogenous, in origin. The further spread through the body, from the portal of entry, takes place in a regular manner and the atrium of infection can almost always be concluded with certainty from the pathological condition of the glands in which the disease is further developed. In the mean, the infection follows the course of the lymph-stream, forming a chain of glands like a row of beads which gets smaller as it approaches the centre. It extends from the place of infection in a circumscribed manner as the process radiates, on account of the numerous anastomosing branches which connect the lymph-vessels one with the other; now and again it extends sideways and sometimes, but rarely, retrogrades.

Bronchial Glands.—It is a well known fact that enlarged and caseous bronchial glands are among the most conspicuous morbid changes observed in tuberculous children, and in necropsies they are almost always found to be involved. So conspicuous indeed are they that up to recent years they have been considered to be the primary lesion of tuberculosis. PARROT, HEDREN, ALBRECHT and GHON have shown that the bronchial gland infections are, in a majority of instances, caused by and consecutive to an initial lesion located in the lungs.

Glands May Calcify.—The mediastinal glands may be involved secondarily to tuberculosis of the sternum, ribs and vertebræ, clavicle or mammary gland. Some writers hold that the entrance of tubercle bacilli into the lymph in any part of the body may cause tuberculous bronchial glands. The bronchial nodes on the right side are more frequently and more extensively involved but it is not uncommon for both sides to be affected. Calcified scars indicate that it is possible for the lesions to become quiescent but in childhood calcification is rare. In the diseased glands caseous degeneration is commonly observed. Only part of the gland may be affected, but when tuberculosis has been the cause of death the whole gland is usually caseated. The caseous mass is surrounded by fibrous tissue which adheres strongly to neighboring organs. When swollen, the glands encroach upon and cause compression of surrounding structures, giving rise to various pressure symptoms. Bronchial glands occasionally suppurate. When they soften they may burst into the mediastinum or form adhesions with and discharge into neighboring organs or on the surface of the chest. They may open into the trachea, a bronchus, the œsophagus, pleura, pericardium, or erode a large vessel. The latter event may cause fatal hemorrhage.

Cervical Glands.—The cervical glands are the most common site of external glandular tuberculosis. The submaxillary group and the nodes along the internal jugular vein are the ones most often involved. The glandular enlargements are usually more extensive on one side than on the other. In the initial stages the glands are firm in consistency, and the individual nodes can be felt. They gradually increase in size and may remain discrete, but more commonly periadenitis binds the glands together in irregular masses. Subsequently there is caseation and softening. Inflammation within the gland is followed by inflammation in the surrounding tissues which results in adhesions or in abscess formation. The abscess may be confined within the gland or involve the surrounding tissues. The skin ultimately becomes adherent and the abscesses, unless opened, burst and leave sinuses which heal slowly and leave disfiguring scars. In other cases the pathological process advances more slowly and a greater amount of fibrous tissue is produced. The glands in such instances are tough and hard and the capsules are greatly thickened. They less frequently form adhesions to the surrounding tissues,' and suppuration is uncommon. Calcification of the cervical glands is rare.[78]

As has been shown under pathogenesis, the tonsils serve in a great number of cases as portals of entry for the tubercle bacilli. Macroscopical manifestation of the conditions is, as a rule, wanting; microscopical study of the tonsil, however, reveals the tubercles situated near the deeper portions of the crypts, and also directly beneath the surface mucosa. These are the most common situations; they may sometimes be located deep in the tonsil close to the capsule. The tonsils may be small and submerged, hypertrophied or of medium size.[79]

Mesenteric Glands.—The changes which the mesenteric glands undergo when infected with tuberculosis, differ in no way from those met with in lymphatic glands similarly involved in other parts These tuberculous nodes are from one-half to one inch in diameter, occasionally larger; from the fusion of several of them may result tumors of considerable size. Primary lesions in the lymphoid structures of the intestine may, or may not, be present. The usual termination of such glands is in calcification; rarely an abscess forms which may discharge into the bowel or into the peritoneal cavity, giving rise to a tuberculous peritonitis. Localized plastic peritonitis is found in all marked cases and may lead to adhesions. '

The usual pathological changes are observed in the inguinal, axillary and other glands when they are tuberculous. In rare instances a generalized tuberculous adenitis occurs.

Tuberculous Lymphangitis.—Although the lymph-channels leading from one lymphatic structure to another are often tuberculous this is usually lost sight of in the general involvement of the tissues. In connection with tuberculous intestinal ulcers and mesenteric glands little crops of tubercles may often be seen in the lymph-vessels of the intestinal serosa. The lymph-channels in the mesentary, in such cases, may become occluded and distended with chyle. Rarely the cutaneous lymphatics become diseased, especially those of the forearm, following tuberculous infection of the fingers. Cutaneous nodules then result which may break down and cause ulcerations of the skin. Tubercles may grow into the thoracic duct or tubercles in its vicinity may rupture and their contents flow into the duct and lead to general dissemination of the bacilli and miliary tuberculosis.

Amyloid Degeneration.—In cases of long standing tuberculous adenitis with chronic suppuration, amyloid degeneration often occurs. It consists in the formation of deposition, primarily in the ground substance of the blood-vessels and connective tissues and especially in the middle coat of the smaller arteries, of a homogeneous appearing albumoid substance. The spleen, liver, kidneys, intestines and stomach are the organs most commonly affected. The amyloid substance shows characteristic staining reactions, e. g., a mahogany brown color is imparted to it by iodine solution. Amyloid disease is quite persistent, but it may undergo surprising improvement in childhood if the primary condition is relieved.[80]

CHAPTER VI

SIGNS AND SYMPTOMS

Tuberculous adenitis has several characteristics which are of interest. The local character of the disease is a prominent feature. The cervical, bronchial or mesenteric glands may be alone involved and only in rare instances is general tuberculous adenitis noted. The local character of the disease is, however, no longer looked upon as a localized expression of a diathesis, but as a distinct evidence of a tuberculous infection. This local characteristic of the disease is not accidental and calls one's attention to the common portals of entry of infection, the respiratory and gastro-intestinal tracts.

The course of the disease is chronic, the lesions persisting over a considerable period of time. The struggle between the infective agent and the protective forces of the lymphatic glands is a long one. There is a tendency to spontaneous healing, the protective forces being sufficient as evidenced by the frequent finding of calcified remnants of bronchial and mesenteric glands. However, the infection may persist for a long period of time and break out afresh and result in an acute tuberculosis.

At the present time this endogenous mode of infection, occurring in later life as a result of intercurrent conditions of disease or unfavorable environment and lowered resistance, is regarded as the most probable source of clinical tuberculosis in the adult. Tuberculous adenitis has thus assumed a position of importance; the recognition of this fact has a most important bearing upon the question of prophylaxis. Tuberculous adenitis is met with at all periods of life, and may be noted even in old age, but is much more common during childhood and early adult years. The most common time of occurrence is between the first dentition and the time of puberty. EDWARDS [1] states that 68% of the glandular adenopathies are observed during the first ten years of life. The question of sex incidence is of lesser import. Most observers are agreed that females preponderate. In WOHLGE-MUTH's [2] series of 430 cases, 223 were females and 207 males. In the author's series of 270 cases, 109 were males, and 161 females.

Bronchial Glands.—The bronchial glands are subdivided into the following sub-groups: [3]

1. The tracheo-bronchial glands, situated in the lateral angles between the trachea and bronchus on each side. Their afferent vessels come from the other groups of bronchial glands and adjacent parts of the trachea and bronchi. The efferent vessels pass to the broncho-mediastinal trunk.

2. The lymph-glands of the bifurcation located in the angle between the two main branches. They are nine to twelve in number and drain the adjacent parts; they also receive the afferent vessels of the broncho-pulmonary glands; their efferent vessels pass to the tracheo-bronchial glands.

3. The broncho-pulmonary glands are embedded in the hilus of the lung and drain the lung substance directly or through the pulmonary glands; their efferent vessels may go directly into the tracheo-bronchial glands or via those of the bifurcation.

4. The pulmonary lymph-glands are situated in the lung substance which they drain; the efferent vessels pass to the broncho-pulmonary glands.

In tuberculosis of children, the bronchial glands are the most frequent site of localization and are almost always involved. This is evidenced by post-mortem findings. In NORTHRUP's [4] series of autopsies on tuberculous children, these glands were involved in 100% of the cases, and in 61% of cases in adults. The nodes on the right side are more frequently and extensively involved than those on the left. WOLLSTEIN [5] found the largest nodes on the right side in 14% of cases. It is not uncommon for both sides to be affected. We have seen that the bronchial nodes are a common site of latent infection which may be dormant and inactive for years, giving rise to no clinical manifestations. In fact, at post-mortem there may be no pathological evidence of

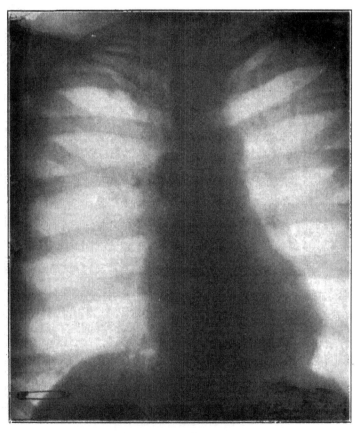

PLATE VII.—Tuberculosis of the bronchial glands in an adult. From X-Ray
Laboratory of Maximilian J. Hubeny, M. D.

infection, it being demonstrable only by animal inoculation. Infection of these glands therefore frequently eludes clinical recognition. They are in relation to the trachea, bronchi, œsophagus, superior vena cava, vagus and recurrent laryngeal nerves. When greatly swollen they may be in contact with the arch of the aorta and the innominate veins. The symptoms and signs are those of pressure upon these structures, together with the toxic symptoms characteristic of a chronic tuberculous process. In a great many instances slight involvement causes no symptoms. In a majority of cases the symptoms are not marked. While children with tuberculosis of these nodes are usually delicate, such is not always the case.

General Symptoms.—The early symptoms are toxic in origin and vary in intensity with the degree of the toxemia. The onset is generally insidious, the condition passing very gradually, often imperceptibly from one of health to that of disease. Disease of the glands may have progressed to a considerable extent before the child, for it occurs most often in children, is known to be ill. Lack of evident cause for change in the general condition is truly characteristic of tuberculosis of the tracheo-bronchial glands, and it certainly is of more frequent occurrence without any special symptoms than with them.

Nervous Manifestations.—The general condition gradually becomes undermined, leading to an irregular and indefinite state of ill health. An early symptom is a sense of undue fatigue after ordinary exertion, often languor and lassitude. With a decrease in strength, the child becomes irritable, restless and fretful and his sleep is disturbed. In older individuals the depression and irritability may advance, until it reaches a condition of typical neurasthenia.

Gastro-intestinal Disturbances.—The appetite may be lost or capricious, and these patients often show a marked aversion to fats. More or less digestive disturbances are frequent. In the early stages, hyper-acidity may be present and later sub-acidity. The nutrition gradually becomes impaired. In well marked cases the child may stop growing or be undersized. Anæmia develops slowly and pallor of the face and mucous membranes may appear so gradually that it is not noted, until it has existed for some time. The reduction of hemoglobin and chlorosis may be a masked tuberculosis. The leucocytes may be normal or show a slight increase. In uncomplicated tuberculosis a leucopenia is not uncommon. Disturbances of the body temperature are a result of the absorption of the toxic products of the tubercle bacilli. Fever is not a prominent feature in tuberculosis of the tracheo-bronchial glands. There is no characteristic type, and many are free from temperature. In incipiency, there is an increase in temperature only after exertion, and it subsides to normal after an hour's rest.

Temperature Changes.—The temperature is more apt to be low in the morning and may reach 99 or 99.5 degrees F. in the afternoon, the rise being slight but regular. Very often the temperature is sub-normal and may be so constantly or increase at night. In a few more active cases, there are long febrile periods in which the temperature is found to be raised more or less continuously. In tuberculous children an increase in temperature is easily excited. Sweating at night may be noted, but is of little significance as it is frequent in children even under normal conditions.

Pressure Symptoms.—When the tracheo-bronchial glands become enlarged to an appreciable extent, symptoms may be produced from pressure upon or irritation of neighboring structures. A spasmodic, metallic, non-productive cough is often the first symptom to excite suspicion of disease of these glands. In young children it may occur in severe paroxysms resembling pertussis. It is not a constant symptom, and I have seen cases in which the glands had reached a large size with practically no cough. Dyspnœa may be a marked symptom especially in infants and younger children. It is most commonly expiratory in character. In spite of it, the voice or cry is clear, showing that it is not laryngeal in origin. It is due seemingly to pressure on the vagus or directly on the trachea and bronchi. Schick [6] thinks that compression of the trachea and bronchi occurs more frequently than is usually stated. He also observed that the dyspnœa was more apt to be present when the child was resting quietly, and that a hard attack of coughing or a disturbance would cause it temporarily to disappear.

Dyspnœa of inspiratory character may result from pressure on the recurrent laryngeal nerve due to paralysis of the dilators of the larynx. Hoarseness, or aphonia, laryngospasm, and asthmatic attacks may also occur.

Sometimes more or less constant pain within the chest is complained of. It is rarely definitely located but is usually in the mid-thoracic region. It may be sharp and lancinating in character and be brought on by deep breathing or exertion. Severe pain may be felt in the region of the upper dorsal vertebræ. Pressure upon the large intra-thoracic veins results in congestion of the mucous membrane of the respiratory tract. As a result, epistaxis and the expectoration of small amounts of blood are not uncommon occurrences. STOLL [7] regards hemorrhage without evidence of cardiac or pulmonary lesions as due to bronchial node enlargement.

Tachycardia is frequent and is probably due in large part to pressure upon the vagus although the direct effect of the toxins upon the heart muscle is a factor to be considered. Pressure of the enlarged glands may cause difficulty and pain in swallowing.

Physical Signs. Inspection.—Individuals with tuberculous infection of the tracheo-bronchial glands may show, on inspection, no particular evidence of it and be well nourished. If the tuberculous infection has been active for some time, however, general signs and symptoms may be noted. These general signs were formerly looked upon as indications of a predisposition to tuberculosis, but are to-day regarded as evidence of an infection, which is flooding the system with toxins.

The trained eye appreciates the general appearance of these individuals. Children are often tall for their age, or at least appear to be on account of the disproportion between the width and height of their chests. Their long slender necks enhance the effect. The fingers are long and thin and the distal digits may be club-shaped. The skin is apt to be dry and scaly and loss of flesh is indicated by its laxity. The hair is often soft, thick and luxuriant, the eyebrows well marked and lashes long and silky.

A special type of facies, "tuberculous facies," has been noted, the face oval in outline, the features delicate and pinched and the expression wistful. The eyes are bright and appealing and the sclera bluish white. The pupils are often dilated, indicating pressure by the enlarged glands upon the sympathetic. When of unequal size the process is more active on the side showing the greater dilatation.

The posture in standing is relaxed, the chest long and often stooped and its circumference subnormal. The scapulæ are situated low and are projecting and prominent. The acromial end of the clavicle is sunken and the shoulders converge anteriorly. The sternum may be arched forward to a slight extent.[8] In most severe cases long continued laryngospasm may so interfere with the entrance of air into the lungs that the anteroposterior diameter of the chest becomes prominent. In older children there may be seen the so-called hilus dimple, a depression visible in the second and third interspaces near the parasternal line when the breath is held at the end of inspiration.

A tracery of enlarged venules interweaving across the chest is a common sign of glandular pressure.[9] They are most often seen in the second interspace between the border of the sternum and the inner half of the clavicle; less commonly they are found in the first and third interspaces also. The enlargement is usually greater on the right than on the left side. When the tracheobronchial glands become greatly enlarged they cause pressure upon the superior vena cava and one or both innominate veins. With great obstruction to the return of blood from the head, the superficial veins may be visible in the temples and neck as well as over the front of the chest. There may be a certain degree of cyanosis of the face, and the skin has a bluish tinge, especially about the mouth. There may also be œdema with puffiness of the lips and eyelids. The cyanosis and œdema are usually intermittent and when only one innominate is involved may be more or less limited to one side of the face.

Palpation.—PETRUSCHKY [10] called attention to the tenderness, on pressure, over the mid-thoracic region posteriorly. It is found in children and adults when the toxic symptoms are

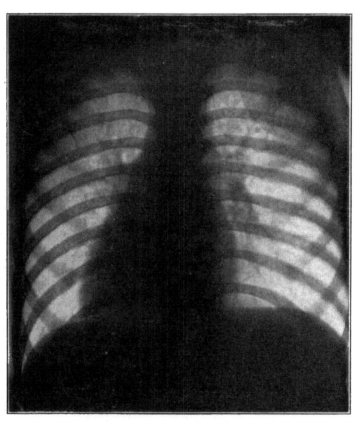

PLATE VIII.—Tuberculosis of the bronchial glands in a child. Age 12 years. From X-Ray Department, Children's Memorial Hospital, Chicago. Kindness of Coleman G. Buford, M. D.

marked, but is not found in latent cases or advanced stages of tuberculosis. Palpation often reveals the pressure of enlarged glands in the cervical region In fact, tuberculous bronchial glands may be demonstrated by the Roentgen Ray in cases of cervical adenitis in which they were giving rise to no symptoms and unsuspected.

Percussion.—Demonstration of enlargement by percussion is a very difficult procedure. They lie deeply and on first consideration it would seem quite unlikely that they could be thus detected. It is only in the event of considerable and extensive enlargement that dulness can be demonstrated. I believe that percussion is of value in such cases if sufficiently delicate.

To percuss the chest posteriorly the patient should be seated on a stool or table with the arms crossed over the chest to the opposite shoulders. The head is flexed forward to secure relaxation of the spinal muscles. A delicate percussion stroke upon the finger of the opposite hand held firmly against the chest wall is employed. I emphasize the fact that the percussion stroke must be light. A tapping stroke will elicit dulness, which is imperceptible when greater force is used, by reason of the inclusion of resonant lung tissue within the percussion sphere. RIVIERE [11] states that there exists normally on either side of the spine, between the first and fifth dorsal vertebra and extending one inch from the mid line, an area of slightly impaired resonance demonstrable by gentle percussion. Another observer believes he is able to detect a normal area of dulness at the root of the lung opposite the fifth dorsal vertebra, the area being slightly larger on the right than on the left.[12]

With enlarged bronchial glands the impaired resonance may extend outward two or three inches from the mid line and may extend down to the sixth or eighth dorsal spine. RIVIERE lays much stress upon this dulness, which is most marked on the right side at the level of the fifth or sixth dorsal spine.

Vertebral dulness is less frequent than paravertebral. In adults a dull note is normally present over the first four dorsal spines. A distinctly dull note below the fourth dorsal is abnormal and may indicate enlargement of the tracheo-bronchial glands. In young children a resonant note is heard over the fourth and not infrequently over the third dorsal spine.[13] It is much less common to obtain dulness from the bronchial nodes anteriorly. When the nodes about the right bronchus are of considerable size, it is sometimes obtained in the second interspace to the right of the sternum. If the tracheal glands are much enlarged, dulness may be found in the first interspace near the right sternal margin and over the right half of the manubrium. Dulness may also be noted along the left sternal margin as low as the base of the heart and great vessels. A tympanitic note may be found over the apex denoting relaxation of the lung. According to various observers the glandular enlargement does not of itself account for all of the dulness. NAGEL [14] believes that there is an actual lessening of lung tissue by displacement. KRAMER [15] believes that enlargement of the mediastinal blood and lymphatic vessels, as a result of obstruction at the hilus of the lung, is responsible for a considerable amount of dulness since the Roentgenogram shows the glands to be smaller than the area of impaired resonance indicates. Another thinks the stasis insignificant and the inflammatory condition of the hilus structure to be the chief factor.[16]

Auscultation.—Auscultation is a valuable and a more trustworthy method of examination. As the bronchial glands become enlarged the vesicular quality may occasionally be replaced by bronchial breathing. It is heard more clearly posteriorly in the inter-scapular space and more often on the right. It is less high pitched and more metallic than the tubular breathing of consolidation or cavity formation. Anteriorly increased vocal resonance is normal over the manubrium. With swollen glands anterior to the trachea and bronchi, whispered bronchophony is marked. Fine râles are sometimes heard external to the hilus in the region of the nipple, usually at the end of inspiration. They are not removed by cough or deep breathing. Pressure of the nodes on the trachea may cause a loud stridor. Loud venous murmurs may be audible, probably due to pressure upon the left innominate vein. This is the basis of Eustace Smith's sign [17] which is elicited as follows.

Eustace Smith's Sign.—The patient is seated in an upright position and directed to extend his head backward upon his shoulders so that his face is turned upward. With the stethoscope placed upon or at the side of the manubrium sterni, a venous hum is heard which varies in intensity according to the size and position of the glands. As the chin is slowly depressed again the hum becomes less distinctly audible and ceases shortly before the head reaches its normal position. According to Smith, the explanation of the phenomenon appears to be that the retraction of the head tilts forward the lower end of the trachea. This carries with it the glands lying in its bifurcation, and the left innominate vein is compressed where it passes behind the first bone of the sternum. He believed the sign to be very reliable evidence of disease and enlargement of the glands, and stated that the experiment failed in healthy individuals. In cases of simple flat chest and enlarged thymus, the latter being in front of the vessels, fixation of the end of the trachea and immobility of the glands would lead to failure in the production of a murmur. Opinions vary as to the value of the sign, some believing it to be of value, and others as unreliable.[18, 19]

d'Espine's Sign.—Some years ago d'Espine [20] called attention to the fact that in children whispered bronchophony normally ceased at the level of the seventh cervical vertebra, but that in enlargement of the bronchial glands it extended downward to the upper thoracic spines. This observation has since been known as d'Espine's sign and has proven to be a reliable factor in diagnosing the disease. It is best elicited when the arms are folded well across the chest, the head sharply flexed, and the patient sitting erect. The examiner auscultates posteriorly over the course of the trachea and the patient is asked to whisper "three-thirty-three" or "one-two-three." Young children can be more readily induced to whisper "tree" or other familiar words. In positive cases the final "e" of the last word persists momentarily after the phonation ceases. This post-phonal quality is a significant feature. The whispered voice gives more satisfactory results than the full voice. The respiratory murmur is the least reliable but may give fair results in experienced hands in the case of infants who do not talk or cry. Loud transmission of the vocal resonance as heard over the normal lung does not constitute d'Espine's sign. The transmitted sound must have tracheal timbre. d'Espine's observations were made chiefly on infants and children. In older children and adults the bifurcation of the trachea is at a lower level than in the infant and, for this reason, the bronchophony is of questionable significance unless heard at a lower level. Opinions differ as to the exact point. FRAZIER [21] believes the sign unreliable unless heard below the level of the first or second dorsal in a child of eight, and below the level of the third or fourth dorsal in a child of twelve. MORSE [22] considers the sign positive, when the bronchial sound extends below the first dorsal spine. HOWELL [23] accepts as a positive d'Espine a change in the character of the whispered voice or expiration at or below the second dorsal.

In a few cases did he find the change as high as the seventh cervical, and frequently as low as the third dorsal without cause. FISHBERG [24] states that transmission of the whispered voice at the level of the third vertebra in a child of ten may not mean enlarged glands in the chest. The intensity of the transmitted sound varies with the position of the glands and the degree of their enlargement. Both the tracheal and hilus glands, when enlarged, may give the sign. The area over which the whispered bronchophony is heard varies greatly. Sometimes it is limited strictly to the vertebral spines but usually it extends to one or both sides. STOLL [25] states that frequently it is heard as far as the left border of the scapula, and quite often it follows the line of the left bronchus. Its import is increased, when heard at one or both sides of the spine as well as over the spinous processes.

Course of the Disease.—The signs and symptoms as above stated may be almost entirely wanting with tuberculous infection of the bronchial glands. When present they are variable and may appear suddenly and remit unaccountably. Children thus affected "catch cold" easily and in ordinary cases severe symptoms may be seen only at such times. In young children they may then become alarming, but their violence usually abates.

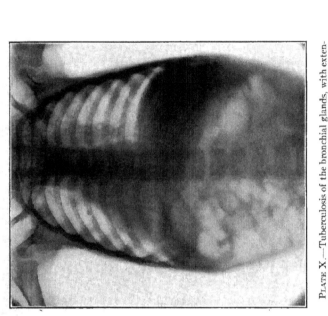

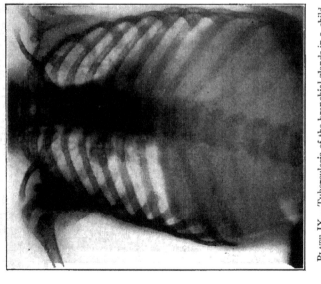

PLATE IX.—Tuberculosis of the bronchial glands in a child. Age 2 years. From X-Ray Department. Children's Memorial Hospital, Chicago. Kindness of Frank S. Churchill, M. D.

PLATE X.—Tuberculosis of the bronchial glands, with extensive hilus infiltration in a child. Age 6 months. From X-Ray Department. Children's Memorial Hospital, Chicago. Kindness of Henry Frederic Helmholz, M. D.

Complications.—The course of bronchial node disease is chronic. That the majority of the glands heal is evidenced by the finding at post-mortem of fibrous and calcified remnants of the nodes in individuals dying from old age or intercurrent disease. The presence in the body of lesions containing virulent bacilli is a constant menace, especially in children under five years of age. In them tuberculous processes are active and the lesions progressive. Simple broncho-pneumonia after acute infectious disease may become converted into the tuberculous type. Miliary tuberculosis of the lungs, or of the entire body, may result from the bacilli gaining entrance to the blood-stream. Tuberculous meningitis is common in children and the tracheo-bronchial nodes are often the source of infection. In rare instances, the glands may soften and rupture into adjacent organs. Rupture into the trachea gives rise to severe suffocative attacks. The alarming dyspnœa may be relieved by the expectoration of a cheesy mass, or the attack of subsequent ones may prove fatal. Fatal hemorrhages into the air passages have been described. The pleura and pericardium may be involved in tuberculous inflammations. Rupture into the œsophagus is an uncommon event. Traction diverticulæ of the gullet may occur from extension of the inflammation from the glands, with adhesions and subsequent cicatricial contraction.

CERVICAL GLANDS

· Tuberculosis of the cervical lymphatic glands is more readily recognized than disease of the bronchial nodes, the affected glands being more superficially located and permitting, when enlarged, of palpation and inspection. Of the external glands the cervical are most often affected with tuberculosis—93% of WOHLGE-MUTH's cases were infected.[26] In TREVES'[27] series of 155 cases they were involved 145 times, and the only seat of disease in 131 instances. Tuberculous adenopathy of these glands is infrequent in infancy. It is most commonly observed during the second decade, but is not infrequently found in adults.

Order of Group Involvement.—The glands in the submaxillary triangle and those of the superior deep cervical group located laterally in the neck along the carotid artery and internal jugular vein are the most frequent sites of infection. Less commonly the supra-clavicular, occipital, pre-auricular, submental and parotid groups are affected. Both sides of the neck are usually involved, but as the disease progresses the more advanced changes are confined to one side in a majority of cases.

Slow and Painless in Development.—The enlarged nodes are at first the only signs. They almost always develop slowly and painlessly during a course of weeks and months. They are first noted as indolent lumps apparently incapable of further change, appearing first in front of, or behind the Sternomastoid muscle at the level of the hyoid bone or upper border of the larynx. In rare instances the onset is acute, the glands enlarging rapidly with more or less pain and temperature. After the subsidence of the acute symptoms the glandular swelling remains and may suffer little or no diminution in bulk. The enlargement of the glands is intermittent. They often increase for a time and then remain stationary, or they may diminish in size. They may take a new start and show further enlargement following inflammation of the associated mucous membranes, acute infections such as measles, or influenza, or simply from deterioration of the general health. As the condition progresses the glands may become as large as walnuts. At first the nodes are separate and discrete and can be felt as individual tumors with smooth capsules and of firm consistency. Adjacent glands become infected until an entire region is involved in many cases, or the process may be confined to a few glands. Eventually they become adherent to each other and become attached to adjacent structures by cicatricial tissue forming irregular knotted masses of large size in which it may be difficult to make out, by palpation, the individual nodes. The course is chronic, the conditions persisting for months, often years. The enlargement may cease at any time, become latent for a longer or shorter period, and again increase or dwindle and disappear spontaneously. Eventually caseation necrosis occurs and later softening.

Suppuration.—HOLT [28] states that of cases allowed to run

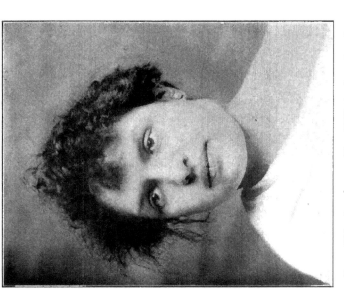

PLATE XII.—Same case as Plate XIV, showing tuberculous involvement of the lymphatics on the opposite side.

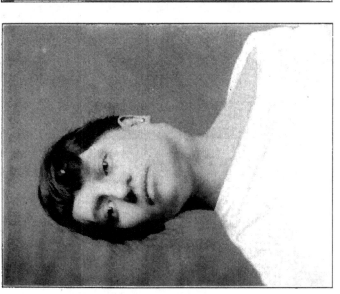
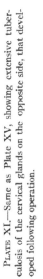

PLATE XI.—Same as Plate XV, showing extensive tuberculosis of the cervical glands on the opposite side, that developed following operation.

their course probably 50% terminate in suppuration. This is followed by inflammation of the surrounding tissues and the skin finally becomes adherent. The abscess may be limited to the gland with a small area of softening, or the surrounding tissues may be involved with more extensive inflammation. Finally the purulent material is discharged through the skin, this process being repeated with the softening of successive glands. The pus is thick and curdy and may be sterile or be proven to be tuberculous by animal inoculation. If secondary infection has occurred, the pus is more like that of an ordinary abscess and the offending organisms can be demonstrated by culture. Where abscesses are allowed to open spontaneously, large irregular sinuses and ulcers result, the condition of the skin referred to as scrofuloderma. There is an indolent purplish patch of skin which is pierced by one or two sinuses or in some instances is riddled by them. The skin lesions are due to a chronic inflammation surrounding the suppurating tuberculous focus. There may be suppuration of the skin from secondary infection with pyogenic organisms, and in rare instances there may be tuberculous ulcers of the skin due to a secondary tuberculous infection. The edges of the ulcers are undermined and ragged. Beneath the skin is an indurated mass in which are embedded numerous caseous and purulent glands.

Sinuses communicate with the glands by a narrow opening, and often continue to discharge for many weeks and months especially when the general condition is poor. These sinuses are notoriously chronic. If a cicatrix forms before the gland is completely discharged it soon breaks down again. If healing occurs a white, puckered disfiguring scar results, as is so often seen about the neck. But suppuration does not necessarily occur. In many cases, if conditions are favorable, the glands gradually diminish in size and return to normal dimensions or remain as small, hard, fibrous nodules. Calcification of the cervical glands rarely occurs.

Secondary Infection.—Tuberculous glands are subject to secondary infection, especially with the ordinary pus-forming organisms, which leads to inflammatory swelling accompanied by pain and tenderness and the general signs of sepsis. Moderate glandular enlargement is not incompatible with good health in other respects, but if the disease is marked the nutrition suffers. When the glands are large and active there is fever. These patients are usually anæmic, particularly if suppuration is of long standing. Tuberculous cervical glands are frequently associated with coryza, rhinitis, bronchitis, eczema of the scalp and face, conjunctivitis or keratitis, etc. The eczema, the catarrhal inflammations of the mucous membranes, plus the enlarged glands, pallor and disturbed nutrition, constitute the picture formerly known as scrofula but now known to be the result of a tuberculous process and its associated toxemia.

Progress Slow and Tedious.—The progress of tuberculous cervical adenitis is usually slow and tedious. Many long standing cases recover. There is a tendency for the inflammation to subside spontaneously about the time of puberty, and cure sometimes follows intercurrent illnesses such as facial erysipelas or scarlet fever. Death rarely follows but may occur in aggravated cases from sepsis, exhaustion and amyloid changes, or more commonly from tuberculosis elsewhere, as in the lungs. In young children these glands may serve as the source of a generalized infection.

The palatine or faucial tonsil has, in recent years, received marked attention for the rôle it plays as portal of entry for the tubercle bacillus in cervical adenitis. Clinical manifestations of tuberculosis of the tonsil are, as a rule, entirely missing. The presence of a tuberculous tonsil can be suspected clinically only by its effects, namely, infection of the tonsillar lymphatic glands.[29] The tonsils may be hypertrophied, small and submerged, or of medium size.

MESENTERIC GLANDS

Tuberculosis of the mesenteric and retro-peritoneal glands was formerly known by the name of abdominal scrofula or tabes mesenterica. We now know that the symptoms included by these terms were due more to the associated conditions than to the infection of the glands, which was often an insignificant part of the disease. Pathologically tuberculous infection of these nodes is common, caseous or calcified nodes being frequent at autopsy and the latter often being found in Roentgen examination of the abdomen. But disease of these nodes of itself rarely causes symptoms, which point to their involvement, and unless there are complicating conditions it may pass unnoticed or be discovered at operation for other conditions.

Usually a Secondary Infection.—The glands are most commonly infected secondarily to tuberculosis of the intestines. However, they may be primarily infected, as it has been demonstrated experimentally in animals, and clinical experience often supports the view, that tubercle bacilli can pass through the intestinal mucous membrane without producing a lesion there, and infect the adjacent nodes. Such infection is analogous to that of the cervical nodes which may be infected without evidence of a tuberculous process in their tributary mucous membrane. Although found most commonly in children it is not confined to them and may occur in adults as well, infection frequently occurring from swallowed sputum, in those who are suffering from a pulmonary tuberculosis. The infected glands become enlarged ordinarily from one-half to one inch in diameter. A number of the glands may become fused together, forming masses of considerable size. Caseation is the usual termination of the glands; less frequently they become calcified and rarely they suppurate.

Often no Characteristic Symptoms.—Except when the glands form masses large enough to be palpable, there are no symptoms which are characteristic or distinctive of their tuberculous infection. Slight enlargement may be consistent with good health. If they remain as the sole lesion the individual's nutrition may remain good, his temperature normal, and slight pallor of the face be the only indication of ill health. In some cases there are no symptoms even with the presence of palpable glands. When there are such symptoms as wasting, diarrhœa, night sweats and increased temperature, they are probably due more to other tuberculous lesions than to the glandular involvement. With intestinal involvement the condition is more serious and the symptoms may be severe. With ulceration there are repeated attacks of diarrhœa with profuse, fœtid, watery stools, often containing blood. The severity of the diarrhœa depends on the extent of ulceration.

Metabolism Impaired.—Intestinal absorption is greatly diminished with resultant loss of weight, emaciation and a coincident loss in strength. The child becomes pale and anæmic, the skin dry and wrinkled. The temperature is increased above normal The rise is usually periodical and more or less in proportion to the degree of intestinal irritation The intestines are often distended with gas and the abdomen tympanitic. The abdominal wall becomes thinned and softened and tender to the touch. In a considerable number of cases the peritoneum becomes involved. In the miliary type of tuberculous peritonitis, there is gradual loss of weight and strength and the abdomen slowly becomes distended with fluid. In the ulcerative and fibrous types, there is a lesser amount of fluid and in addition adhesions which bind together the glands, intestines and omentum. The abdomen becomes distended, on palpation it is tender and firm, and large nodular masses of glands or adherent intestines and omentum may be felt. On percussion checker board dulness may be elicited; this is a very valuable diagnostic sign. Intestinal obstructions or fecal fistulæ may result.

Localized Involvement Stimulating Appendicitis.—The glands in the ileocæcal region may alone be involved and give rise to symptoms simulating appendicitis. There may be tuberculosis of the appendix and cæcum, or the glands may be infected primarily. An analogy is to be noted between the infection of the glands adjacent to the appendix and infection of the cervical glands adjacent to the palatine tonsil. The appendix is a lymphoid structure and has been called the abdominal tonsil. In such cases abdominal pain having an acute onset, accompanied by nausea and sometimes by vomiting, may become localized in the right iliac fossa. Local examination reveals tenderness and rigidity of the abdominal muscles but a tumor mass is rarely palpable There may be repeated attacks of such pain, simulating very closely appendicitis Although it may appear to be somewhat atypical of appendicitis, unless the patient shows well-marked evidence of tuberculosis, a differential diagnosis may be impossible until the abdomen is opened at operation. Such cases have been reported by GAGE, EISENDRATH, PARKER and others.

Local Manifestations.—Many cases of tuberculosis of the mesenteric glands show dilatation of the superficial veins of the abdominal wall. In exceptional cases the glands may be large enough to press upon surrounding structures. Pressure on the vena cava may cause œdema of the legs. Ascites may be due to enlarged glands in the hilus of the liver with pressure upon the portal vein. Pressure on the nerves may result in cramp-like pain in the lower limbs. Unless they are considerably enlarged the mesenteric glands are not palpable, when sufficiently enlarged they may be felt on deep palpation as irregular masses at the sides of the spine at about the level of the umbilicus. Enlarged glands may occasionally be reached by rectal palpation.

Softening of the glands is infrequent. When it occurs it may lead to a localized abscess among the intestinal coils, or may ulcerate into the intestines. Of the uncomplicated cases, perhaps a certain and not small proportion recover under suitable treatment, even when the glands were large enough to palpate. In such cases recovery depends largely on the treatment. With complications the course is downward, with intestinal ulceration, diarrhœa and wasting, or more often by an outbreak of tuberculosis elsewhere, as a meningitis or miliary tuberculosis.

TUBERCULOSIS OF OTHER LYMPHATIC GLANDS

Frequency.—Lymphatic glands of the body, other than the bronchial, cervical and mesenteric, are less often infected with tuberculosis, as is to be expected, on account of diminished exposure. The following statistics are indicative of the frequency of their involvement:—[30]

	Balmann's findings	Wohlgemuth's findings
Neck and occipital	81 %	93 %
Axillary	6 o %	2.78%
Inguinal	7 o %	.93%
Popliteal	o7%	.23%
Cubital	5 o %	23%
Auricular	— .	2 9 %

The Axillary Glands, from eight to ten, to fifteen or more in number, are situated in the axillary space and drain the mammary region and side of the thorax, both the superficial and deep areas. Although less frequently observed than cervical node involvement, tuberculous infection of these glands is by no means rare. Not infrequently they are infected in connection with the cervical glands. The most common sources of infection are tuberculous lesions of the arm and hand, tuberculosis verrucosa cutis, or anatomical wart, received through injury at autopsy or otherwise, and tuberculosis of the mammary gland. The glands may not be affected in the former conditions, but they generally are found to be involved in tuberculosis of the mammary gland. The diseased nodes are felt as firm movable nodules in the soft tissues of the axilla. They may reach the size of walnuts, but they do not often lead to the formation of abscesses and sinuses.

The Cubital Glands are not invariably involved in infections of the hand and fingers, but tend to become infected in deep processes. They may, in such instances, be diseased in conjunction with the axillary glands, or be alone infected.

The Inguinal Glands.—Tuberculous infection of the inguinal glands, although far from common, is more frequent than is generally recognized. The infection may be derived from several sources and the primary focus may not be evident. It is not infrequent in connection with tuberculous lesions of the genitalia about the anus or within the pelvis. HOLT [31] and others have reported cases of tuberculous inguinal adenitis following circumcision, the wound being infected by the operator. Tuberculous ulcers resulting from wounds of the feet may be the source of infection. DOWD [32] has reported such cases.

The infection attacks both the deep and superficial glands.

The femoral nodes in Scarpa's triangle and the inguinal groups along Poupart's ligament become involved and the infection exhibits a tendency to spread upward into the pelvis, through the lymphatic structures, surrounding the iliac vessels. Involvement of the nodes may be rapid or slow, and the infection virulent or very mild.

The Popliteal Glands are rarely involved in a tuberculous infection and when observed it is secondary to infection of wounds of the feet.

GENERALIZED TUBERCULOUS ADENITIS

A rare occurrence is a tuberculosis of nearly all the lymph-glands of the body with little or no involvement of other parts. It occurs more often in negro patients and in connection with pulmonary tuberculosis. It is usually accompanied by a temperature of 101 to 103° F. and the course of the disease is often rapidly fatal Any or all of the superficial gland groups, cervical, axillary, or inguinal, may be involved. The glands are firm and caseous and may be greatly enlarged. There is often extensive involvement of the bronchial, mesenteric and retro-peritoneal glands. There may or may not be active tuberculous lesions elsewhere.

Differentiation from Hodgkin's Disease.—The more acute cases resemble Hodgkin's disease very closely. In infants and children the infection may involve various groups of glands in succession, more rarely simultaneously. Such cases are usually fatal, death being due to a meningeal infection, or cachexia, and exhaustion.[33]

TUBERCULOUS LYMPHANGITIS

Tuberculous lymphangitis is a rare occurrence, if we exclude those cases in which mesenteric lymphatic vessels are involved in connection with a tuberculosis of the intestines, and can be traced through the mesentery to the receptaculum chyli, and the involvement of the thoracic duct in miliary tuberculosis. In rare instances tuberculous lymphangitis develops in the ex-

tremities, more often in the upper, in connection with tuberculous lesions of the fingers, such as tuberculous ulcers or sinuses,
which have followed the rupture of an osteal focus.

The Lymphatic Vessels.—Small firm nodules develop along
the course of the lymphatic vessels. When numerous they may
form a cord-like infiltration. The nodules slowly increase in
size and may undergo caseation and softening and discharge
externally leaving ulcers and fistulæ. A provisional diagnosis
of tuberculosis of the deep lymphatic vessels may be made if an
abscess, which has no connection with bone or joint, develops
in the course of the large lymphatic vessels.[34]

CHAPTER VII

PROGNOSIS

The progress of tuberculosis of the lymphatic system depends upon many factors, the most important of which are the extent of involvement, resistance to infection, virulence of same, and age of patient. Many other factors, of course, have a bearing on the question, for instance, the social position which still plays quite an important rôle in determining the sentence of life or death amongst our infants.

Any factor that tends to lower the resistance of the patient ought to be considered when prognosticating a tuberculous condition. Lack of proper food, unhygienic surroundings, and malnutrition have a decidedly unfavorable influence upon the course of tuberculosis. The importance of these factors can never be overestimated.

The age of the patient is undoubtedly the most predominating factor from the standpoint of prognosis. The younger the child, the graver the outlook. If a child can be protected from a massive infection up to 7 or 8 years his chances for life are very much improved.

The virulence of infection determines to a large extent the course of the disease. Bovine infection is, as a rule, mild in its course and yields readily to proper care. The virulence of the human type bacillus varies markedly from a very mild affair to the fulminating types.

The extent of involvement and regions involved are apparent in their importance. The more extensive the involvement, the worse the prognosis, and the more vital regions involved, the more dangerous the condition. Bronchial gland tuberculosis is more serious than mesenteric glandular involvement and cervical adenitis.

Bronchial Gland Tuberculosis.—The prognosis in this condition is always serious but far from fatal. The majority of children having infection of the bronchial glands recover, when they are placed in good surroundings and treated properly. The younger the child, the more grave the prognosis. Involvement of the bronchial glands in babies under one year usually means death, between one and two years recoveries are less exceptional. From three on the prognosis is more and more favorable. Observation teaches us, says HUTINEL,[1] that the majority of children carried away by miliary tuberculosis (meningitis) have caseous foci in their bronchial glands, and the softening of these foci seems often to have been the cause of the final explosion.

As the child grows older the frequency of latent tuberculosis increases and chances for recovery are now much better if correctly treated. But there is one more period of life that is quite important and acquires its annual toll, namely, the period of adolescence. Boys between 17 and 20, and girls from 14 to 16, often fall an easy prey for the enemy trenched in amongst the bronchial glands.

The size of the lesion will not lend itself to prognostication because the gravity of the condition is independent of the size of the glands. Large masses may recede, sclerose and heal up, while the small active foci may be the cause of rapidly fatal complications, especially meningitis.

The presence of pulmonary lesions in active state have an important bearing upon the question of prognosis. Modern pathology teaches us that the great majority of cases of hilus tuberculosis is due to a pulmonary infection, the focus, however, often being so small that a painstaking search is required to find the same. A great many of these youngsters succumb to the first attack, a certain number rally, however, having the hilus infection as a remembrance of their former struggle. A secondary infection of the lungs now, from the bronchial gland focus, constitutes most probably the ordinary type of adult tuberculosis The younger in life it occurs the correspondingly graver is the situation.

Several intercurrent diseases manifestly play an important rôle in awaking latent foci of bronchial gland tuberculosis. Measles and whooping cough are universally known often to be followed by manifestations of active tuberculosis. Many children having weathered successfully the acute infections succumb to a tuberculous complication, e. g., meningitis Post-mortem examinations in these cases often reveal softened caseous foci in the bronchial glands. The modus operandi in these cases is self-evident. The bronchial infection always present in measles and whooping cough overtaxes the diseased lymphatic system of the lungs. The walled-off focus becomes suddenly the seat of pronounced inflammatory changes, the localized tuberculous lesion becomes disseminated, parts of the same may enter the blood-stream, and a miliary tuberculosis result.

Mesenteric Gland Tuberculosis.—Simple involvement of the mesenteric glands, without any intestinal complications, is not a very serious matter. Most of these cases recover under proper management.

Complications, however, may change the entire outlook. Rupture of an enlarged gland causes tuberculous peritonitis which may, however, under favorable conditions go on to recovery.

Tuberculous ulcers of the intestine, as a rule secondary to pulmonary tuberculosis, often represent the last stages of the disease. Sometimes these patients may be kept alive for a year or two, but this is, as a rule, a sorrowful existence due to the marked diarrhœa and subsequent emaciation.

Tuberculous Cervical Adenitis.—Tuberculosis of the external lymphatic glands *per se* may have a fatal outcome. Secondary infections may produce a marked toxic condition due to the prolonged suppuration which, together with poor resistance and malnutrition, may cause death. But tuberculous cervical adenitis is, as a rule, called to our attention before such a condition exists, and nearly all these cases will respond to proper treatment.

When suppuration and sinuses are already present the prognosis of complete recovery must be somewhat guarded. But wonderful results are obtained at the present time under proper management. Tuberculin and X-Ray stand forth as the most important remedial agents. Personally, I have by means of tuberculin caused many tuberculous sinuses to heal with only slight scar formation.

The rational use of tuberculin has a marked influence upon the prognosis of tuberculous lymphadenitis. Our experience coincides with that of BANDELIER and ROEPKE in that we have never seen a gland break down under tuberculin treatment. Similar results have been obtained by many men. It seems to the author that a remedy, which in the hands of many different men has met with so wonderful success should, at least, get part of the recognition it deserves from the profession at large.

CHAPTER VIII

DIAGNOSIS

CLINICAL DIAGNOSIS

Tuberculosis of the Bronchial Glands.—The clinical picture of tuberculosis of the bronchial glands is by no means distinct, and rarely is the entire symptom complex present and pointing to the diagnosis. The early symptoms especially are indefinite. The recognition of physical signs of disease of these glands is difficult, and often unsatisfactory because of their situation deep within the chest. In the early stages there may be no physical signs although the disease is active. In attempting to make a diagnosis, therefore, no line of investigation should be omitted and all possible information which might be of value obtained.

Importance of Care in Taking History.—A history should be carefully taken as it may give important data. Inquiry is made as to the existence of tuberculous disease in the parents, or in other children in the family, or in associates, with whom the patient comes in close and frequent contact. The presence of tuberculous disease in the parents does not, as was formerly supposed, point to hereditary predisposition or predestination to tuberculosis in the child, but is of great importance since it serves as a source of infection. It is during early life that contact between children and their parents or associates is closest, and it is at this time that susceptibility to infection is greatest. Inquiry should be made as to the occurrence of previous diseases, and especially concerning a recent attack of measles, whooping cough or influenza. An allergic state occurs in such conditions as is demonstrable by the negative v. Pirquet test in children in whom it had previously been positive. These diseases are important in that they may be the etiological factors in the activation of a previously latent infection. A prolonged and unsatisfactory convalescence from such disease should always lead one to think of tuberculosis.

Insidious Onset.—In discussing symptoms, I called attention to those symptoms and signs constituting the general picture of the disease. These are in large part toxic in origin and must not be overlooked. The insidious onset, with feeling of languor and fatigue, the anorexia or capricious appetite, the neurasthenic symptoms, the loss of weight and impaired nutrition, the pallor, the slight rise in temperature, are all general symptoms observed in early tuberculosis.

But any or all of these symptoms may be present from causes other than tuberculosis. Bearing this in mind other factors should be excluded. Thus anæmia, fatigue and malaise are symptoms which may result from overwork in school, late hours, lack of fresh air, digestive disturbances, and other conditions, as well as from tuberculosis.

Temperature.—Too much attention must not be attached to a slight rise in temperature in children, for in childhood it is a frequent occurrence from such causes as infection of the naso-pharynx or accessory sinuses, pyelitis or digestive disturbances. Such things should be thought of and eliminated.

Cough and Dyspnœa.—A dry cough may be due to naso-pharyngeal irritation or enlargement of the lingual tonsils. The cough in tuberculosis of the bronchial nodes resembles closely that of pertussis. The latter, however, more often shows nightly exacerbations and the paroxysms are more frequently accompanied by vomiting or the expectoration of mucus. If these conditions can be excluded the cough is quite diagnostic. The dyspnœa frequently observed, when there is pressure on the bronchi or trachea, resembles that of laryngeal croup except that the voice is not lost.

Asthmatic attacks in children should always lead to suspicion of bronchial node tuberculosis.

Spinalgia.—The spinalgia described by PETRUSCHKY is present with active inflammation, but is not found with cheesy nodes. The tenderness may be slight or very acute, and unless definite it is of no value. To judge the degree of tenderness note the facial expression while palpating over the spine. De La CAMP noted this sign in 87% of 100 incipient cases. The spinalgia disappears with rest in bed and tuberculin. Cardiac disease should be eliminated, as spinal tenderness may occur with it. The tenderness noted in neurasthenia, in contradistinction to that of tuberculosis of the tracheo-bronchial nodes, is not limited to the upper thoracic vertebræ

Spinal Dulness.—On percussion of the vertebral spines from above downward the sound is dull and the tactile resistance exaggerated over the upper three or four dorsal vertebræ, below which level the remaining thoracic spines afford low pitched resonance with a distinct osteal quality. Dulness extending down to or below the fifth or sixth dorsal vertebra is pathologic. This may be due to bronchial glands, when they are considerably enlarged. Aneurism of the aorta, mediastinal neoplasm, consolidation of the lung, pleural effusion and a dilated heart may cause spinal dulness, and should be thought of, and ruled out as possible causes when diagnosing glandular enlargement.

d'Espine's Sign.—I consider d'ESPINE's sign of great value in diagnosis. The transmission of the whispered voice indicates that some tissue, denser than normal, is present between the trachea and bronchi and the anterior surface of the vertebral column, which transmits the sound without modification. While it shows nothing as to the character of the tissue, experience shows that it is usually glands. A positive d'ESPINE sign has a great value. When it is negative it must be remembered that tuberculous glands may be present, but not enlarged to a sufficient extent, or so situated as to be interposed between the trachea, bronchi and the vertebral column. The sign is regarded as of value ,by STOLL, DAUTWITZ, SMITH, BACH and others. While the control of the sign by autopsy has not been large, cases have been observed by d'ESPINE, STOLL and others. I consider EUSTACE SMITH's sign of little value.

Neisser's Pressure Method.—NEISSER proposed to test the sensitiveness of pressure of tuberculous bronchial glands by means of a distensible sound introduced into the œsophagus.

He made use of a hollow sound with a rubber finger cot tied over the fenestra. By means of a rubber bulb this could be inflated at various levels and pressure thus exerted on the glands from within the œsophagus. Tenderness was elicited in cases of tuberculous glands, while healthy individuals were free from pain. Though ingenious, the method is little used.

Tracheo-Bronchoscopy.—In some cases tracheo-bronchoscopy has been made use of. The bulging of enlarged glands, lying near to the trachea and bronchi, may be recognized. Because of the difficulty encountered in diagnosing tuberculosis of bronchial glands, all signs and symptoms should be looked for. A single sign or symptom cannot make a diagnosis. "The presence of dilated veins, spinalgia, dullness and d'Espine's sign, speaks for enlarged glands." Their tuberculous nature is practically assured when, in addition to these, the individual is under weight, has a paroxysmal cough and symptoms of toxemia.

X-Ray.—The use of the X-ray in the diagnosis of tuberculosis of the bronchial glands, is of considerable value. Enlarged and pathological glands can often be demonstrated by this means, when the symptoms are general and vague, and the local symptoms and physical signs are altogether wanting. The X-ray may show gland involvement, when they have not yet reached sufficient size to cause cough, dyspnœa or other pressure symptoms, and when they are too small to cause a d'Espine's sign or appreciable dulness. Studies of the X-ray, percussion, or d'Espine's sign, show them to be of about equal diagnostic value.

Steroscopic Plates.—In the examination of the chest by means of the X-ray, we may use the fluoroscope, a single plate, or the steroscopic plates. The latter are always preferable, since they show the shadows in perspective, and enable the observer to appreciate the third dimension, and the depth of the lesions from the surface of the chest. Shadows are visible in steroscopic plates, which are not in single plates, in which they are superimposed. While the fluoroscopic method of examination is of great value, the plate method is preferable. In an X-ray plate, we have a permanent graphic record of the varying density of the tissue through which the rays have passed. The fluoroscope, on the other hand, is an observation but not a record, and gives us nothing tangible for further study or comparison.

Normal Findings.—In the radiograms of a normal chest the bony skeleton with its covering of soft parts stands out plainly, the ribs bounding the chest on all sides, except the narrow inlet above, and below where we have the diaphragm. Within the chest several groups of shadows may be seen and are described as the central opacity or shadow, the hilus shadow, and the markings in the lung fields.

Interpretation of Radiograms.—The central shadow is large in size and distinct. It is made up of the shadows cast by the vertebral column and the mediastinal contents, consisting of the heart, aorta, and other great vessels, œsophagus, trachea, lymphatics, and connective tissue. The trachea can often be distinguished, as a light band bounded on either side by darker bands, and its bifurcation at the level of the fifth dorsal may be visible.

The Hilus Shadow.—The hilus shadow is noted at the level of the fifth, sixth and seventh dorsal vertebræ. Normally it is of moderate density, of small extent and irregular in outline. It is caused by the density of the primary bronchi, the pulmonary vessels and their contained blood, and the lymphatic and fibrous tissues of the hilus of the lung. Toward the median line it merges with the heart shadow, but on the right it is distinctly seen extending outward into the lung field. The outer margin of the hilus shadow is irregular, because of the shadow cast by the bronchial, and vascular trunks extending outward from the hilus into the parenchyma of the lung.

Lung Markings.—In the lung fields we find the linear markings; near the hilus they are heavier and more distinct than toward the periphery. In some plates the shadows may be seen in groups corresponding roughly to the lobes of the lungs as the shadows extend toward, but not quite to the periphery of the lungs. These markings are, like the hilus shadows, made up of the shadows cast by the divisions of the bronchi, the blood-vessels and their contained blood, together with the accompanying lymphatic vessels and fibrous tissue. The intensity of the markings is greater in adults than in children.

Early Tuberculous Changes are noted by an increase in the area and density of the hilus shadows These changes are due to an increase in the fibrous and lymphatic tissue which accompanies a mediastinitis. But such changes may be caused by infections other than tuberculosis. The finer markings may be more prominent and appear broader, denser and extend closer to the periphery of the lung. The lines may be studded, or broken in continuity and show a delicate network.

Normal Glands Cast no Shadow.—In early involvement the individual glands may not be seen, the only thing noted being an increase in the width of the lung root. When the glands become caseous they appear as more or less shadowy spots. Calcified glands are sharply defined and easily recognized. When a large mass of nodes is present a distinct lobulated mass may be seen. Shadows can be diagnosed as glands only when they are more or less homogenous, and of well defined margin Since the central opacity may obscure glands on the left side, plates should be taken in an oblique position, the rays passing from behind on one side to in front on the other. In this way the spinal column, heart, and great vessels will be seen separated by clear space, unless diseased glands are present in the mediastinum.

X-Ray Diagnosis not Easy.—Diagnosis of disease of the bronchial glands by means of the X-ray is not an easy matter. The skiagram should be taken and the plates interpreted by a specialist, skilled in this line of work.

Even when glands which cast shadows are found, one is not assured by the X-ray plate that he is dealing with an active tuberculosis. The X-ray is thus of value only when the clinical findings are used in conjunction with it. Upon our clinical findings must we base our opinion, that the glandular enlargement is due to tuberculosis by excluding other conditions, which might cause an enlargement of these glands. Likewise we must depend upon clinical observation in basing our opinions as to the activity of the lesions. Calcified glands, which show most distinctly on the X-ray plates, tend to indicate a lesion which is undergoing healing. DUNHAM and WOLMAN [1] state that the presence of calcified glands, other conditions being favorable, may be taken as a good prognostic sign.

TUBERCULOSIS OF THE CERVICAL GLANDS

As a rule tuberculosis of the cervical glands presents little difficulty in diagnosis. The suspicion of tuberculosis should be entertained in every case of chronic enlargement of these glands. The location of the swellings, their slow course without apparent cause in most instances, and the presence of large masses of glands bound together by adhesions, all point to tuberculosis. The chronicity and comparative absence of symptoms is of much importance in diagnosis.

The tendency to caseation and suppuration is characteristic, and when the glands have ruptured and indolent discharging sinuses and puckered scars exist, the diagnosis is relatively easy. The formation of fistulæ, the thin fluid secretion containing caseous fragments, and the usually long standing, indicate the tuberculous nature of the lesions, while thick yellow pus, an acute course, marked inflammatory symptoms, and early scarring, indicate a different origin. While the onset of the enlargement is at times acute, the persistence of the increased bulk of the glands, after the subsidence of the acute manifestations, should lead one to think of tuberculosis.

Must be Differentiated from the Following Diseases.—Tuberculosis of the cervical glands must be differentiated from a number of conditions, causing chronic glandular enlargement in this region.

Syphilis is a common cause of enlargement of these glands. In the early stages of syphilis the glands of the groin, axilla and epitrochlear regions are affected. Later the glandular involvement is more extensive. In the neck the glands of the posterior cervical region are more distinctly indurated, while in tuberculosis the anterior chains are most often affected. Suppuration of these glands is rare. There may be a history of syphilitic infection, or concomitant signs of syphilis may be present. A positive Wasserman blood test may be obtained. The glandular enlargement subsides under anti-syphilitic treatment.

In Lymphatic Leukemia the cervical glands may be enlarged. Anæmia develops more rapidly than in the tuberculous infection. The blood examination clears up the diagnosis, the large number of white cells and the presence of myelocytes being pathognomonic.

Pseudoleukemia or **Hodgkin's disease,** may require differentiation. In the early stages the cervical glands alone may be enlarged. Sooner or later other groups are involved. The disease is rare in children, being most commonly observed in adult males. The posterior cervical and the supra-clavicular groups are most often affected. Less often the submaxillary or anterior cervical. The glands are more freely movable and less sensitive than tuberculous glands. Their consistency is uniform, and they do not caseate or suppurate. In doubtful cases the diagnosis can be established by excision of a node and microscopical examination.

With tuberculous nodes the X-ray examination may show spots of calcium salt deposits. Although not commonly found it is very characteristic of tuberculosis when noted.

Cysts.—Large solitary glands may resemble cysts. In favor of cysts is their location in the neck in a position typical of these structures. The presence of smaller nodes immediately surrounding these, speaks for tuberculosis. In doubtful cases the test puncture, or an examination after excision, settles the diagnosis.

Malignancy.—In old age solitary glands must be distinguished from malignancy. They should lead to a search for a primary malignant lesion, and in doubtful cases the diagnosis should be made positive by excision and microscopical examination.

Sarcoma of the lymphatic glands is to be distinguished by the more rapid enlargement of the nodes, and the early involvement of the adjacent tissues.

Actinomycosis rarely causes difficulty in the diagnosis. The sulphur granules made up of the ray fungi, found in the pus, are diagnostic.

Tuberculosis of the Mesenteric Glands

Tuberculosis of the mesenteric glands frequently runs its course without pressure symptoms or functional disturbances, its only indication being general symptoms such as increased temperature, pallor and loss of weight. Abdominal pain and watery offensive stools, due to the associated intestinal condition, are suggestive.

Tuberculosis of these glands can be diagnosed with certainty, when the glands are palpable. Considerable enlargement is necessary, before they can be felt. Palpation is often hindered by flatulent distension or fæcal accumulations. Deep palpation in the region of the umbilicus may detect firm or movable masses on either side of the spinal column. One must assure himself that the bodies felt are not masses attached to the omentum, or lumps of hardened fæces. The former are more superficial and consequently more easily felt than glands and are more freely movable. Fæcal masses are elongated and of moderate size with their long axes in the direction of the bowel and they are situated at some place along the colon. They are not deeply placed and are more easily reached than glands; they can be indented by firm pressure. In case of doubt, fæcal masses are easily removed by a copious enema or by a cathartic, while masses due to any other cause are made more evident. Enlarged glands can occasionally be felt by rectal palpation.

Percussion will often manifest checker-board dulness, this may be difficult to determine in inactive cases of tuberculous enlargement of the mesenteric glands, but is more easily shown when there is activity in these glands, with its accompanying inflammatory exudative changes, and is a valuable diagnostic sign. It may be an aid in determining activity. This sign may also be present in tuberculosis of the intestines, mesentery or parietal peritoneum.

Tuberculosis of Other Lymphatic Glands

The Axillary Glands.—The diagnosis of tuberculosis of the axillary glands is rarely difficult. The chronicity and persistence of the infection and the association with tuberculous cervical glands, tuberculosis of the mammary gland, or with a tuberculous affection of the hand, arm or forcarm, indicates the nature of the lesions.

The Cubital Glands.—Tuberculous cubital glands likewise can be diagnosed with ease when there is a tuberculous lesion in the area tributary to these glands, which is the evident source of infection. Enlargement of the epitrochlear glands is common in syphilis, and in the absence of a local infection and a recent acute general infection, is considered by many as pathognomonic of lues. Glandular enlargement due to lues will respond to antisyphilitic treatment.

The Inguinal Glands.—Tuberculosis of the inguinal glands is often mistaken for a complication of some venereal disease, at least until its stubbornness, chronicity and resistance to treatment arouse a suspicion of tuberculosis. Since venereal diseases, and especially syphilis, are the most common cause of inguinal adenopathy, they should be thought of at once and eliminated. Careful examination of the patient may reveal a tuberculous lesion of the genitalia, or of the feet, which is the source of the glandular infection. In cases where it is very desirous to eliminate Hodgkin's disease, or a possible malignancy, a gland may be excised for microscopic examination or animal inoculation. A large tuberculous gland in the inguinal or femoral region may simulate the appearance of a hernia.

The Popliteal Glands.—What has been said in regard to the diagnosis of other glands will apply to the popliteal nodes. The chronicity of the infection and the presence of a lesion, which serves as the source of the infection, are the most important points. Although tuberculosis of the popliteal glands is rare, as statistics show, it should not be forgotten.

SPECIFIC DIAGNOSTIC METHODS

Tuberculin Diagnosis.—"Tuberculin is the most exact and finest reagent for proving the existence of a tubercular deposit, in the living organism." [2] The result of tuberculin reactions have not fulfilled the greatest hope that was built upon them, following the announcement of their application in the specific diagnosis of tuberculous lesions. But they do have a definite value and have thrown much light upon important questions in tuberculosis, especially as an aid in making an early diagnosis of tuberculosis, also in determining the time of the infection, and the great prevalence of latent infections; they, therefore, merit careful consideration. In using tuberculin for diagnostic purposes we may make use of the cutaneous tests, including that described by v. Pirquet, the intracutaneous and percutaneous reactions, the conjunctival test of Wolf-Eisner or the subcutaneous test.

Different Tests.—In the cutaneous tests the tuberculin is introduced into the superficial lymph spaces of the skin, and does not gain access to the blood-stream. The interaction, occurring between the immune substances and the tuberculin, liberates the toxins from the tubercle bacillus protein contained in it and this occasions the inflammatory reaction at the site of application. In the subcutaneous test the tuberculin gains access to the blood-stream, and in a sensitized individual gives rise to a general reaction with a rise of temperature of a variable extent, constitutional symptoms of toxæmia, and a focal reaction at the site of disease which may cause an exaggeration of the signs and symptoms recognizable clinically. In addition, there is a local inflammatory reaction at the site of application of the tuberculin to the subcutaneous tissues. For a discussion of the theories of the tuberculin reactions see chapter on Tuberculin treatment.

CUTANEOUS TUBERCULIN TESTS

v. Pirquet's Test.—The cutaneous test of v. Pirquet is one of the most extensively used and is a valuable tuberculin test, being easily performed and harmless.

The site usually chosen is the inner side of the forearm because of its delicate and less hairy surface and the ease of observation. In children the outer aspect of the arm may also be employed. The skin is first cleansed with alcohol or ether and quickly dried by evaporation. Two drops of Koch's old tuberculin are then placed about four inches apart. The skin is stretched taut and scarified by means of a chisel-shaped instrument made for the purpose, a needle, or the point of a scalpel, first at a point midway between the drops as a means of control, and then in the drops themselves. The scarification should be but deep enough to open the superficial lymphatics of the skin, any considerable oozing of blood to be avoided as in vaccination. The scarifier should be heated before use to remove any tuberculin that may be present from a previous test as this would cause a reaction at the site of control. The tuberculin is allowed to dry for several minutes and the excess is then removed with a bit of cotton.

Positive Reaction.—The slight inflammatory reaction incident to the trauma soon abates. The true reaction usually makes its appearance within twelve to twenty hours after the application of the tuberculin. On rare occasions it appears within four to six hours. The extent of the reaction varies. In mild reactions there is slight redness and infiltration, while in more severe types the redness covers a more extensive area, and the infiltration results in a well-marked papule from three to twenty mm. in diameter. The reaction reaches its height in twenty-four to thirty-six hours, and the inflammation then subsides. The patient experiences only slight pain or itching; general reaction and fever, as well as focal reactions are almost invariably absent, although they have been observed.

In rare instances the latent period exceeds twenty-four hours, and reaction phenomena are sometimes delayed four or five days. Such late reactions occur in clinically unsuspected cases and only exceptionally in manifest tuberculosis. In a negative reaction the points of inoculation appear like the control. It requires some experience to distinguish minimal reactions from traumatic or negative ones. v. Pirquet recommends that the beginner regard as doubtful all reactions under five mm. in diameter and to repeat the test. Now and then the first test is negative, and an intense reaction occurs when it is repeated.

Reaction Due to Hypersensitiveness.—The test depends on the hypersensitiveness of the skin of the tuberculous person to the small amount of tuberculin taken up by the lymphatics. The test may be considered as specific in demonstrating hypersensitiveness due to the presence of a tuberculous focus. It does not, however, offer an accurate indication as to the state of activity of this focus, unless other factors are considered. Histological examination of excised papules shows nodular masses of epitheloid cells, partly surrounded by a zone of round cells, the typical giant cells of Langhans and distended capillaries, the picture of typical tubercles without caseation changes such as are caused by toxins of the tubercle bacillus.[3]

The test has been applied in a very large number of cases. It is important in that it has permitted the recognition of latent foci and given information as to the great frequency of tuberculous infections and the time of its occurrence.

Frequency of Infection.—The following table given by VEEDER and JOHNSON [4] shows the frequency of infection according to age as determined by the v. Pirquet reaction:

Age	St. Louis Veeder and Johnson	Vienna v. Pirquet	Hamburger
Under 1 year	1 5%	0%	0%
1–2 "	5.5%	0%	9%
2–4 "	19%	13%	26%
4–7 "	25%	30%	54%
7–10 "	30%	38%	75%
10–14 "	36%	70%	94%

In Adults of Little Value.—A positive v. Pirquet reaction gives us no information as to the site of the tuberculous disease. Those who are clinically tuberculous and the non-clinically or anatomically tuberculous give a response. These facts limit to a very great extent the diagnostic value of the reaction in adults; a positive reaction affords us no practical conclusion as to treatment. v. Pirquet did not regard this method as appropriate for use in adults. In them it must be subservient to clinical manifestations of disease. When distinctly positive and accompanied by considerable infiltration and erythema about the site of application of the tuberculin, a thorough examination and careful observation of the patient is imperative.

Great Value in Children.—In young children the test is of greater importance since it enables the time of infection to be determined. The younger the child the greater its value. In sucklings a positive reaction proves the presence of active tuberculosis, and a negative reaction the absence of infection. In older children, as in adults, many who react are clinically healthy, possessing only small inactive foci.

We may conclude—

1. That the cutaneous test is specific.

2. That the cutaneous reaction is almost invariably positive when tuberculosis is present except under certain well defined conditions.

3. That the test may be negative in case of acute miliary tuberculosis, tuberculous meningitis, the terminal stages of pulmonary tuberculosis, and in acute infectious diseases as described below.

All reactions occurring in young children should be regarded as suspicious. A negative test in a child under ten years, carefully performed, excluding advanced tuberculosis or a recent attack of measles or other acute disease, is as good evidence as can be obtained that the condition is non-tuberculous. On the other hand, a positive test in a child over six years must not be estimated too highly as evidence of clinical tuberculosis.

Degree of Reaction as a Guide.—The degree of reaction is no guide to the extent of a tuberculous process but may be indicative of the degree of resistance, and the quantity of immune bodies possessed by the individual and with certain limitations may give information as to the state of activity of the lesions. Thus in active disease the body cells react and produce larger quantities of free circulating antibodies. Such cases usually reach a maximum cutaneous reaction within twenty-four hours. In disease which is healing and approaching quiescence it may be assumed that there are fewer circulating antibodies, and the maximum is reached subsequent to twenty-four hours. In healed cases the reaction occurs late and is slight. In attempting to compare the v. Pirquet reaction with clinical manifestations it is to be remembered that, on the basis of the latter, different observers will draw different conclusions as to the state of activity of the disease.

Pottenger's Views.—POTTENGER [5] has made a study of the test in regard to its availability as an index of the state of activity of a tuberculous focus. In drawing his conclusions he considers points in the history indicative of the activity of the disease, the physical signs, the condition of the muscle, noting spasm or degeneration, and any diminutions in motion of the diaphragm as shown in a limitation of motion of the side of the chest. Positive active lesions showed uniformity in reaction. I quote the following from him—"It (the reaction) usually came on early, manifesting itself even as early as six hours in some cases. In most cases, however, where it was given in the afternoon the reaction would be found in the morning on the patient's awakening. This would increase in severity during the next day reaching its maximum before or about the end of the twenty-four hours. It would remain at its height for a short time and then gradually disappear. Aside from the reaction coming on soon in these early active cases, it was usually well marked. In those patients where I had given an opinion that there was a latent lesion, I usually found that, while the reaction might be in evidence the following morning and keep increasing during the first twenty-four hours, it would probably not reach its maximum until the second day and in some instances even the third. The reaction in these cases was also quite marked but the principal thing I noticed was that it did not come on so early. In the border-line cases we had variations between these two reactions. A reaction might come on early but keep increasing after the first twenty-four hours. It was, as a rule, not a marked reaction when a case was practically healed. When we could find no evidence of anything but an old lesion with no clinical symptoms and nothing to indicate activity, as a rule we had a very slight reaction on the day following the inoculation, which rarely increased to any extent." From a study of forty-four cases of suspected early pulmonary tuberculosis, the clinical history, physical examination, condition of the muscles and the v. Pirquet taking the twenty-four hour limit as indicative of activity, they agreed in 76.2% of cases giving a percentage of difference of 23.8%. The clinical history, physical examination and the v. Pirquet based on twenty-four hour limit agree in 78.2% giving a difference of 21.4.%."

POTTENGER further states: "It is possible that the twenty-four hour is not the correct one to differentiate between active and quiescent lesions, but yet, as my cases will show, it was correct in the majority of instances. It makes me at least feel that a v. Pirquet which comes on, reaching its maximum within twenty-four hours from the time the inoculation was given, is indicative of an active tuberculous process. If these results can be confirmed by others the v. Pirquet test may yet be saved to the profession as a means of differentiation between active and quiescent lesions."

From a personal study of ten cases of clinically healed tuberculosis that were active when first observed, but had recovered under tuberculin treatment, five years having passed since any tuberculin was given them, the following findings were observed which are of marked interest. These cases were all subjected to the v. Pirquet test. At the end of twenty-four hours one case gave a slight reaction, which increased, reaching its height at thirty-six hours and was slow in subsiding. At the end of thirty-six hours a slight reaction was present in five more of the cases, and at the end of forty-eight hours there was only a faint trace of these reactions present. At the end of forty-eight hours the remaining four cases gave a very faint reaction, the evidence of which lasted from four to twelve hours.

The clinical history and physical findings at the time of this investigation indicated that there were no active tuberculous foci. In the one case that gave a reaction at the end of twenty-four hours an exhaustive study was made, but there was nothing found to indicate activity. This case was observed for one year and there developed no evidence of any further tuberculous involvement.

The v. Pirquet tuberculin test gave 100% of reactions in these ten cases of clinically healed tuberculosis; 10% reacted at the end of twenty-four hours, 50% reacted at the end of thirty-six hours, and at the end of forty-eight hours 100% had reacted; 90% of the reactions occurred after the "twenty-four hour" time limit. The results observed would tend to confirm the value of a v. Pirquet test as an aid in determining the activity or inactivity of a tuberculous lesion.

As a result of my investigations, I believe that the positive v. Pirquet test must be regarded as of little value in children over three years of age, or in adults, unless the time limit reaction is taken into consideration.

A negative v. Pirquet, in the absence of manifest tuberculosis in either children or adults, is, I believe, definite evidence of the freedom from either a latent or an active tuberculosis.

Tice [6] concludes from his experiments that a negative test in the adult, all circumstances considered, is of more value than a positive one.

Percutaneous Test

Ointment Test.—The application of tuberculin to the skin in ointment form, has been employed for diagnostic purposes by Moro and Doganoff in their percutaneous test. They make use of an unguentum consisting of equal parts of old tuberculin and anhydrous lanolin. The preparation darkens with age but retains its potency for some time. For the test, a portion of the ointment as large as a pea is thoroughly rubbed into the skin for one minute over an area of about five centimeters in diameter. The upper abdomen, or the region about the nipple offers the most favorable site for the test.

Positive Manifestations.—In a positive test there occurs at the site of inunction within twelve to twenty-four hours an efflorescence of papules. They are red in color and accompanied by some erythema of the surrounding skin. They become well marked in twenty-four hours and reach their height in forty-eight hours in a typical response. Their appearance may be delayed in some instances until the third or fourth day. The intensity of the reaction varies with the individual cases. There may be only a few papules, or they may be numerous, closely set and accompanied by inflammation of the surrounding skin.

In most severe reactions they may go on to vesiculation. The reactions are particularly severe in so-called scrofulous individuals, in whom there may be papular eruptions at various places in the skin, in addition to the area which has been anointed with the tuberculin ointment.

I have observed that when the infection involves structures rich in blood supply, such as the skin, the reaction to tuberculin is severe, but if there is a limited blood supply as in the bones, the response is mild. This is undoubtedly due to the fact that in the one instance there is an opportunity for extensive antibody contact, and in the other it is limited.

Test Uncertain.—The test is more or less uncertain. There is a difference in the powers of absorption of various skins. The length of time and the vigor employed in applying the ointment will result in a variation in degree of absorption, consequently in the test there is considerable difficulty in judging the degree of reaction. It is usually judged by the number of papules which appear, and by the extent of the inflammatory disturbance. But since variation may be the result of other factors, the value of the test as an index of the reactivity of the individual to tuberculin is thus limited. The test is of much less value than either the cutaneous or subcutaneous.

The individual making the test will do well to protect with a rubber cot the finger which he uses to apply the ointment. Ordinarily there is no danger, but if the rubbing with the unprotected finger is continued long enough, sufficient tuberculin may be absorbed to cause a local reaction. The test may be employed in the case of children in which there is vigorous objection to the hypodermic injection, or to the scarification for the v. Pirquet. But practically these objections to the other more reliable tests are negligible, and consequently I do not employ the percutaneous test. If made use of, a reaction occurring as described may be taken as evidence of "immune bodies" to tuberculosis, the test being specific. Negative reactions are interpreted the same as for the other tests. Like the v. Pirquet the greatest practical value is in its use in children. There are no contraindications to its use except in case of so-called "scrofulous" children, in whom the reaction may be severe and extensive

Intracutaneous Test. Method Employed.—Mantoux and Roux have described and employed the intradermic injection of dilute solutions of tuberculin for diagnostic purposes. The technique of the performance of this test is as follows:—

The skin of the forearm is chosen as the site of injection and is cleansed with iodine or ether. A sterile glass syringe equipped with a very fine needle is employed for the injection. The skin is stretched and the needle inserted nearly parallel with the surface, with the aperture of the needle directed upward until the point is within, but not through, the skin. One drop of a 1:5000 dilution of old tuberculin is injected. A white elevation of the skin is evidence that the injection is intradermic. A control injection may be made using the diluent.

Local Manifestations.—When the reaction is positive a slight infiltration, perceptible to the sight or touch, is noted in five or six hours. At the end of twenty-four hours the reaction is usually well marked. At the sight of injection there is a red papule which is surrounded by a zone of erythema. The size of the papule varies little, the violence of the reaction being determined by the size of the halo. The reaction is at its height at the end of forty-eight hours, and during the second or third day begins to recede. The peripheral halo first disappears; the papule becomes violet in color, then brownish, and disappears in two or three weeks. If no reaction occurs with the dose mentioned, it may be increased and the test repeated.

No General Symptoms.—The injection may occasion itching, discomfort and sometimes slight pain. There are rarely ever any general symptoms unless the tuberculin is injected in part beneath the skin, when a febrile reaction may occur. When the test is negative there is slight induration and brownish discoloration which disappears in two or three days, at which time a positive reaction would be at its height.

A Delicate Test.—This reaction is probably the most delicate of the cutaneous tests. It is more sensitive than the v. Pirquet, and has the advantage that the amount of tuberculin introduced can be measured. It has the disadvantages of being more difficult to perform than the v. Pirquet and causes more discomfort. In adults its value is limited as in the other tests. By using various dilutions of tuberculin different degrees of reactivity may be noted, and as a means of estimating the degree of hypersensitiveness it has no equal. It is superior to, but less practical, than the v. Pirquet and is applicable to cases where the subcutaneous method is contraindicated.

Conjunctival Test.—Instillations of solutions of tuberculin into the conjunctival sac have been used for diagnostic purposes, and were first described by Wolff-Eisner and Calmette as the conjunctival and ophthalmic tests.

Method of Employment.—The lower lid is gently drawn down and one drop of 1% solution of old tuberculin is gently dropped into the conjunctival sac from a pipette or ordinary medicine dropper. The drop should be allowed to fall gently, and the pipette held near so that the eye is not irritated, and the drop should be immediately expressed by the closing of lids, or washed away by the increased lachrymation. The lid should be held down for a half minute to permit the conjunctiva to be bathed with the solution. A protective dressing may be used to exclude traumatic irritation, but this is usually not necessary. Koch's old tuberculin is used, the diluent being sterile normal saline.

Evidence of Reaction.—A positive reaction is indicated by reddening of the conjunctiva, which appears in six to twenty-four hours. In mild reactions the inner canthus and lachrymal caruncle are the seat of most marked changes. In more severe reactions swelling of the follicles and a flow of tears appear; the ocular conjunctiva and the sclera are also involved, or a fibrous or suppurative secretion is seen with œdema of the lid. Subjectively the reaction resembles an ordinary conjunctivitis, and gives a sensation of a foreign body or a feeling of heat, itching and pain. The inflammatory reaction reaches its maximum in twenty-four to thirty-six hours and then subsides in mild responses, being over in two or three days and in more severe reactions in four to six days.

In case the reaction proves to be negative and it is desired to repeat the test, the tuberculin solution may be used in the same strength or increased to 5% concentration. The test must not be repeated in the same eye since the reaction to a second drop may be alarmingly severe. Wolff-Eisner claimed that the test could be employed without danger, but others are of a decidedly different opinion.

Contraindications.—There are numerous contraindications to the use of this diagnostic reaction. Existing inflammation of the conjunctiva or uveal tract contraindicates its use. CALMETTE and WOLFF-EISNER, however, employed it in the presence of mild conjunctivitis. History of previous eye disease such as phlyctenular conjunctivitis is likewise a contraindication because of the danger of a severe reaction which may prove destructive. It should not be employed in hyper-ergic or manifestly "scrofulous" individuals or in those with skin lesions about the eye suspected of being tuberculous.

Dangers.—Untoward effects may be noted in the aged for in them the impaired nutrition of the cornea may lead to ulceration. Senility and arteriosclerosis, therefore, prohibit its application. Severe and serious eye changes lasting for months have been observed and very severe keratitis, corneal opacity, very acute conjunctivitis with chemosis, ulcers, etc., have occurred from its use, even with the application of fresh tuberculin solutions and the observance of proper technique in every respect.

Wolff-Eisner's Views.—WOLFF-EISNER believed that a positive reaction indicated active tuberculosis, for the tuberculin solution was either quickly absorbed or washed away. Unless a large number of circulating antibodies were present, the tuberculin would be carried away quickly and no reaction would occur. But this belief, that only the clinically tuberculous, or those in danger of an outbreak, respond to the conjunctival test, has not been sustained. It is subject to the same limitations as the other tests and has been observed to be negative in cases of active tuberculosis, and positive in clinically inactive cases. Since the eye is such a delicate and all important organ, and the test not more reliable than less dangerous ones, it is folly to employ it, and it is little used at the present time.

Subcutaneous Test. Most Valuable Test.—The subcutaneous test was the first method employed in the use of tuberculin as a diagnostic measure. It may still be considered as the last resort and most searching method in tuberculin diagnosis, as applied to doubtful or obscure cases of tuberculosis. I prefer its use to that of the various cutaneous methods previously described. BANDELIER and ROEPKE[7] speak of it as the most practically serviceable, and most fertile in results, of the diagnostic methods. In younger children only does the v. Pirquet test suffice, and the subcutaneous test is then applicable to older children and adults.

Accurate Dosage.—In employing this method an accurate dosage of tuberculin is obtained. It is deposited in the subcutaneous tissues and its absorption is thus assured. In addition to the local inflammatory reaction, the tuberculin reaches the bloodstream and is distributed throughout the body resulting in a general reaction. This affords further objective evidence of the reactivity of the body to tuberculin, which is indicative of the presence in the organism of the immune bodies of tuberculosis. The irritation of the focus of infection constitutes the focal reaction, which is absent in the cutaneous tests. The focal reaction often expresses itself clinically by the appearance of symptoms and signs of disease, also the exaggeration of existing symptoms, which may prove of great value in locating the site of an obscure tuberculous focus.

History and Examination Prior to Test.—Before applying the subcutaneous test the other methods of diagnosis should first be employed. The history of the patient should be taken in detail, noting any evidence of tuberculous disease and its course and progress. A thorough physical examination should be made, and the physical signs carefully noted and recorded for purposes of comparison at the time of reaction, and to facilitate the recognition of a focal reaction. The patient should live under the same conditions, during the period of observation preceding the test and the time immediately following, in order that extraneous factors may be eliminated and the reaction, if one occurs, be properly interpreted.

Importance of Temperature Range.—Since the increase in temperature is an important part of the reaction to the subcutaneous test, the temperature should be noted for at least two days before the test injection is given. It should be taken at intervals of two hours and recorded on a chart. In a hospital or sanitarium the temperature may be recorded by a nurse or attendant. If the patient is in the home, or is up and about, he may be instructed as to the keeping of a temperature record. The temperature should be taken accurately, and there are many sources of error. The thermometer should be held in the mouth long enough to register. To insure accuracy, it is necessary to hold the thermometer for two or three times the interval in which it is supposed to register. Thus a one-minute thermometer should be retained two or three minutes. Before taking his temperature, the patient should keep his mouth closed and avoid talking or eating and drinking as these affect the temperature of the mouth for some time. Rectal temperature is more accurate. In the female the menstrual period should be avoided, because of the frequent occurrence of menstrual and premenstrual fever, and also out of consideration for the patient's general health at such time If the patient is to be in bed after the test is given he should likewise be in bed during the days preceding. This is not essential, however, and the test may be applied to patients who are about.

Technique of Test.—Prior to making the subcutaneous test, the temperature must be taken at regular intervals for at least two days to determine the temperature range, as well as the normal for the individual. This temperature range may be as much as 1½ degrees even with the high temperature being at normal or possibly only 99 degrees. A period of subnormal temperature, I have observed, often precedes the febrile period in tuberculosis and is a most important symptom of tuberculosis. The average temperature for the two preceding days may be considered as the temperature for the individual, and must be the base from which the reaction temperature is figured, whether it be afebrile or febrile.

Method Employed.—The administration of tuberculin in the subcutaneous test does not differ from the administration of any remedy by the hypodermic method. Aseptic technique, proper dilution and dose of tuberculin are the essentials to be observed. An all-glass syringe is preferable, since it can be easily sterilized by boiling. Before injection the skin at the chosen site should be cleansed by iodine or ether and allowed to dry by evaporation. The choice of the site of injection is a matter of little consequence. The forearm, arm, lumbar, abdominal and interscapular regions have all been employed. Personally, I make use of the outer aspect of the arm, this being a convenient site for observance, and for injecting the tuberculin into the subcutaneous tissues.

For the subcutaneous test any of the tuberculins might be used, since the protein substance of the tubercle bacillus, the ingredient of tuberculin responsible for the reaction, is present in all of them, although in variable quantity.

Selection of the Tuberculin.—I employ Koch's old tuberculin and this is the one used by the majority of men engaged in work on tuberculosis. Its use is more familiar and more study of it in regard to dosage has been done than with other preparations. Bovine tuberculin is less desirable than human. Sometimes a patient will react to one, and not to the other, or to the two with a different severity of reaction. A reaction to either should be considered positive.

The making of the dilutions is a simple procedure and should occasion no difficulty. If one is using tuberculin for either diagnosis or treatment, he should make his dilutions fresh at the time of injection. For those who do not regularly employ diagnostic tuberculin, proper dilution may be obtained in ampoules. I do not advise the use of the latter, or of tuberculin solutions that have been kept for longer than two weeks, as such dilutions unquestionably become less active and are, therefore, unreliable. The original tuberculin can be kept for many months, even after unsealing the package. This is especially true of

Koch's old tuberculin. Any solution showing turbidity should not be used.

For making dilutions a pipette or glass syringe accurately graduated in tenths of cubic centimeters is essential. As a diluent I use sterile distilled water. To secure proper dosage two solutions should be made. The first is a 1:100 dilution made by the addition of 0:1 cc. of old tuberculin to 9.9 cc. of diluent; 0:1 cc. of this dilution contains 1 mg. (0.001 gm.) of tuberculin. By the addition of a ½% of phenol this dilution will keep for months and can be used for the basis of future dilutions. For the second dilution 0.1 cc. of the first solution is added to 0.9 cc. of diluent. This makes a 1:1000 solution of tuberculin, 0.1 cc. of which contains 1/10 mg. (0.0001 gm.). From one of these two dilutions any desired dosage can readily be prepared.

Time for Injection.—There is a difference of opinion as to the most suitable time for injection. Some prefer giving the dose late at night. On the other hand, others prefer the early morning hours, fearing that the reaction may occur unnoticed if the injection is given at night.

Dosage to be used for Diagnosis.—As in the administration of remedial agents, the dosage of tuberculin injected for diagnostic purposes will vary with the age and vigor of the patient, and with the type of tuberculous lesion. Koch's suggestion was to give at intervals, three doses, a first of 1 milligram, a second of 5 milligrams, and a third of 10 milligrams; the latter dose to be repeated in case of no reaction. By reason of the fear attendant on the use of tuberculin these doses have been considered as too large, and practically all clinicians make use of smaller ones. Personally, I prefer the injection of much smaller doses.

Diagnostic Doses of Tuberculin for the Subcutaneous Test

Age	1st Dose	2nd Dose
Up to 5 years	1/100 mg.	1/80 mg
5 –10 years	1/80 "	1/60 "
10–15 "	1/40 "	1/30 "
15–20 "	1/20 "	1/10 "
Adult	1/10 "	1/5 "

For a child then under five years I begin with 1/100 mg. If

no reaction—focal, general or local—occurs in seventy-two hours, I increase the dose to 1/80 mg. In younger children I stop with the second dose, in older children and adults a third dose may be given which then should be the next larger one in the above scale. For an adult as an average initial dose, I give 1/10 mg. increasing at seventy-two hour intervals to 1/5 mg. and 1 mg. if necessary.

Small Doses Preferable.—I consider these smaller doses as sufficient, and believe that conservatism should be the watchword in the use of tuberculin for diagnostic purposes. Experience teaches me that a vigorous reaction often follows a slight increase in dosage or even the repetition of the same dose, which on a previous administration resulted in no reaction. When larger quantities of tuberculin are injected, the reaction to the repeated and larger doses may be severe, and while I believe no harm ever results from tuberculin when used by physicians experienced in its use, the severer reactions cause considerable discomfort, and I consider a marked rise in temperature as unnecessary. No hard and fast rules can be laid down for the determination of dosage in each individual case. The age and vigor of the individual, and the probable state of activity of the tuberculous lesion must be taken into consideration. One's clinical experience is the most valuable aid in the determination of dosage. Some observers advise the repetition of a small dose without increase. Thus LOWENSTEIN proposed not to increase the dose at all, but to repeat a dose of 2/10 mg. four times in ten or twelve days.[8] Argument has been raised by some against the repetition of dosage on the ground that the reaction following a third or fourth injection is due to the protein instead of a reaction due to the immune bodies resulting from a focus of tuberculosis. WOLFF-EISNER considers this a distinct objection. Theoretically it is possible that anaphylaxis might be caused by the proteins contained in the tuberculin and account for the reaction occurring on subsequent injection without tuberculous infection being present. But the amount of foreign protein injected is so small that the production of hypersensibility in this manner is quite improbable. Those who use this method, however, find that the non-tuberculous react only after many more repetitions of dosage than are necessary to cause a reaction in the tuberculous. For practical purposes, therefore, the dose may be repeated and increased as indicated without detracting from the specificity of the test in indicating the presence of tuberculous infection. From a theoretical standpoint, an initial dose of tuberculin large enough to cause a reaction is to be preferred to repeated smaller doses. But the determination of such dose is manifestly impossible with any great degree of accuracy. Having in mind the avoidance of severe reactions and great discomfort to the patient, smaller doses, repeated as is necessary, are for practical purposes, not only permissible but to be advised. Other observers make use of and advise larger doses than I employ. Thus POTTENGER [9] recommends as an initial dose for an average adult 1 milligram. Two days later, if there is no reaction, he gives 3 to 5 milligrams and three days later, in case of no reaction, 7 to 10 milligrams. BANDELIER and ROEPKE [10] regard an initial dose of 1 milligram as unnecessarily large and recommend that the initial dose be fixed at 2/10 milligrams (0.0002 gm.). If no reaction occurs with the first dose, a second and larger one may be given but not until the lapse of at least forty-eight hours to avoid the recurrence of a late reaction.

Maximum Dose.—It is obviously quite impossible to fix a definite maximum dose for the determination of the presence of tuberculosis or infection, a dose below which the tuberculous individual will react and the healthy will not. The human body is a variable quantity, no two individuals in health being alike, and still greater differences are imposed when conditions of disease exist. Koch recommended as a maximum dose 10 milligrams, which he repeated once for the sake of greater certainty. As with the determination of the initial dose, all factors in any given case should be taken into consideration. An average frequently quoted is 5 milligrams for a child, 7 milligrams for an adult in lowered vitality, and 10 milligrams for a vigorous adult. As previously noted I consider such maximum doses as too large.

The Reaction.—With the subcutaneous test the reaction is fourfold and may be discussed under the following headings:

1st. The febrile reaction, consisting of a rise in temperature to a variable degree;

2nd. The general or constitutional reaction, comprising the toxic symptoms accompanying a rise in temperature;

3rd. The local inflammatory reaction, at the site of injection;

4th. The focal reaction, occurring in the focus of disease.

The Febrile Reaction.—The rise in temperature is the most regular symptom of reaction to tuberculin as applied in this test, and the one commonly depended upon. It can be measured accurately and objectively with the thermometer. A certain interval of time elapses between the time of injection and the appearance of fever or other symptoms. This constitutes the incubation period, and is the time in which the specific antibodies are engaged in breaking up the tubercle bacillus proteid, and liberating its toxic portion.

Time of Reaction.—The time of reaction begins usually 10 to 16 hours after the injection of tuberculin. In rare instances it begins in 3 to 4 hours or may be delayed two or three days. The temperature may show a rise of, only a fraction of a degree, but such should arouse suspicion and be considered evidence of a reaction, if there are concomitant general symptoms or a local reaction. In a mild reaction the temperature reaches 100° F. In severe ones it reaches or may exceed 102° F. The reaction ordinarily reaches its height within 24 to 48 hours after the time of injection and then gradually falls, reaching the normal in 24 to 48 hours except in the most severe responses. The febrile reaction is subject to variation and no typical temperature curve can be described.

Variations in Reaction.—There is usually a more or less rapid rise, followed by a more gradual fall to the normal. In interpreting the reaction, increase of the temperature due to intercurrent infections, menstrual fevers, and the like, must be excluded. In neurotic individuals a febrile reaction may sometimes follow the needle puncture alone. If such is suspected, it may be eliminated by giving sterile water at the first injection.

Constitutional Reactions.—The general symptoms are toxic in origin and resemble those occurring with the toxemia of bacterial infection. The patient suffers from malaise, loss of strength, increased nervousness and anorexia. They feel "achy" and depressed, and complain of headache and soreness in the muscles. In more severe reactions the nervousness is marked, and severe headache, pain in the back and limbs, chills and vomiting may be noted. The symptoms resemble those of the onset of an acute infectious disease. They are usually in proportion to the extent of the rise in temperature, but may be well marked in cases with only a slight or even a negative febrile reaction. In such cases they are characteristic and indicative of a reaction. When the general symptoms are noted and properly interpreted, there is no necessity for the production of such great febrile reactions. The general symptoms usually subside quickly, but in very severe reactions prostration may persist for several days. In such an event the patient should be confined to bed.

The Local Reaction.—The local reaction consists of congestion and infiltration at the site of injection. Like the febrile reaction it varies in the degree of its severity, and usually quickly subsides. In case the temperature is increased only a part of a degree, the occurrence of a local reaction is confirmatory to the doubtful febrile reaction.

The Focal Reaction.—The production of a focal reaction is the distinguishing characteristic of the subcutaneous test. It is also a most important characteristic and one not observed in the other tuberculin tests, which fact gives the subcutaneous test superiority as a diagnostic measure. The focal reaction consists in an inflammatory process in the tuberculous focus with the production of symptoms and signs of disease, thus enabling one to determine the site of infection. In superficial lesions, such as lupus or tuberculous glands, a focal reaction is very evident. When the lesions are situated internally, unfortunately the reactions are often not definite enough to be convincing, and in their absence it cannot be concluded that no focal reaction has occurred. The symptoms will vary with the location and extent of the disease. In order to recognize a focal reaction, a careful physical examination previous to the application of the test is essential.

Negative Reactions.—Negative tuberculin reactions are observed in various acute diseases, notably measles, scarlet fever, influenza and less often in diphtheria, pneumonia and others; negative results are also observed in some cases of manifest tuberculosis, miliary tuberculosis and tuberculous meningitis. SAHLI [11] offers the following possible explanations for such negative reactions:

1. The body may contain such an excess of lysinized tuberculin that the extra amount does not display any action.

2. The tissues may be so damaged that they produce no lysin.

3. The lysin may be so far neutralized that the injected tuberculin finds no free lysin to act upon and, therefore, proves inactive.

Specificity of the Test.—The specificity of the tuberculin reactions, as an evidence of tuberculous infection, can hardly be contested at the present time. The occurrence of positive reactions in apparently healthy individuals, and in various conditions of disease, was formerly considered as evidence against the test as a specific one. The demonstration of the great frequency of latent tuberculous foci by the autopsy findings of numerous observers, leaves little doubt but what a tuberculous infection is present whenever the reaction is positive. Its occurrence in disease, such as syphilis, may be explained by the existence of a focus of infection, since it is not found to be positive in all cases. That positive reactions in leprosy may be due to a group reaction is a very probable suggestion, when we consider the similarity of the bacilli of tuberculosis and leprosy, both in their morphological characteristics and in the type of lesions which they produce. Others have sought to disprove the specific character of the reaction by claiming that reactions may be obtained in tuberculosis by the injection of indifferent substances such as albumen and peptone. But the specificity of tuberculin is to be maintained by reason of the fact that relatively large amounts of these indifferent substances are required to produce a reaction, while minute amounts of tuberculin suffice. The reaction with tuberculin is not due to its albumose content, for reactions are obtained with albumose free preparations.

Dangers of the Test.—The subcutaneous test is held in fear by many by reason of the unfavorable results obtained with the use of tuberculin when it was first introduced. Such unfavorable results must, however, be attributed to its improper use. There are those who consider that the focal reaction, attended by congestion and exudation in the focus of infection, may lead to a spread of the disease. SAHLI [12] in speaking of diagnostic injections says: "I consider the risk attending their use sufficient for their rejection." In contrast to such views is the experience of the vast majority, who have used tuberculin to any extent. All those who have had a wide experience state that when properly administered, tuberculin does not cause extension of the disease. On many occasions have I seen marked improvement following a diagnostic injection, and when given as I have indicated, I have never seen harm result. POTTENGER makes the following significant statement: "The frequency with which patients, who have been suffering from an active tuberculosis, improve following a reaction produced for the purpose of diagnosis will more than offset any supposed harm that might have resulted in other cases. Any one who has had such experience in the employment of the subcutaneous test must have observed this."

Contraindications to the Subcutaneous Test.—There are several contraindications to the subcutaneous test. It is an unnecessary procedure, and because of the discomfort to the patient which it may occasion, it should not be employed, when the evidence obtained from the physical findings or the demonstration of the tubercle bacillus leaves no doubt as to the diagnosis. The existence of fever of 100° F. would mask a reaction and, therefore, contraindicate its use. It should not be used in pulmonary tuberculosis following a recent hemoptysis as the reaction may be negative at such time. Disease of various organs constitutes relative contraindications. We should consider severe valvular lesions, and advanced myocardial degeneration as indications for its non-use. Severe nephritis likewise contraindicates. It should not be employed in cases of miliary tuberculosis, tuberculous meningitis, or during convalescence from severe disease such as scarlet fever, measles, influenza, typhoid or pneumonia, as it may be negative even in the presence of tuberculous infection, and hence could not be of any value. Since it has been known to aggravate cases of epilepsy, it should not be used in individuals so addicted. Severe diabetes and marked arteriosclerosis contraindicate its use. The cutaneous test should be applied in such cases.

Interpretation of Tuberculin Reactions.—In interpreting tuberculin reactions, it must be remembered that a positive reaction is but an indication of the presence in the organism of specific immune bodies, whether they are considered as anaphylactins or lysins. Since these bodies may be present as the result of lesions which are inactive, and constitute infection but not disease, it is evident that the value of the tests must always be more or less relative.

Test May Determine Activity or Inactivity.—I have considered the value of the v. Pirquet test in childhood and its interpretation. In my opinion the subcutaneous test must be admitted to be the superior test in older children and adults from the standpoint of diagnostic value, since in it we know the definite amount of tuberculin introduced and are assured of its absorption. The occurrence of a focal reaction is likewise an important characteristic possessed only by the subcutaneous test. We are interested in tuberculous disease rather than in tuberculous infection. The drawbacks to the usefulness of the tuberculin test lie in its delicacy in indicating hypersensitiveness, and in the fact that nearly every individual has, at some time in his life, had a tuberculous infection. That hypersensitiveness varies must be admitted. My personal experience teaches me that there is a very noticeable difference in the reactions occurring in active disease, and in latent infections. In general we may say that prompt and vigorous reaction to small doses is indicative of active lesions, and sluggish and delayed reactions or to larger and repeated doses indicate latent infections. All who have had much experience with tuberculin must have noted this fact. But there are many intervening degrees of reactivity difficult of interpretation, and the dividing line between active and latent tuberculous foci is by no means sharply drawn. In such cases the occurrence of a focal reaction may be of great assistance, especially in cases with superficial lesions, or in surgical tuberculosis so-called.

Value of Experience With the Tests.—The more familiar one is with the use of tuberculin, the better able one will be to judge reactions, and interpret them properly in the individual case. While admitting the difficulty in interpreting reactions in doubtful cases, I must agree with BANDELIER and ROEPKE when they say—"It would, however, be a crime against the spirit of diagnosis to let what has been said prove an insurmountable barrier to the use of tuberculin in diagnosis."

In case of tuberculosis of superficial glands in which the diagnosis is doubtful, the subcutaneous test may be employed and the occurrence of a focal reaction easily determined. When such occurs the glands show an inflammatory reaction to a variable degree. In addition to the febrile and general reaction the affected nodes become tender to the touch and spontaneous pain may be complained of. In well-marked reactions the glands may become appreciably enlarged. If the skin has become adherent it may become reddened. If sinuses are present, the discharge from them may be increased in amount. With the subsidence of the reaction, improvement usually is noted. This applies to tuberculous cervical glands so commonly noted, and also to infections of the axillary inguinal or other superficial nodes.

Interpretation of Tests.—Latent infections of the bronchial nodes are a frequent cause of positive reactions in those who clinically are non-tuberculous. As noted above, I consider the character of the reactions as an important indication of the activity of the lesion, active lesions responding promptly and reaching a maximum early, while less active or latent infections result in reactions which respond less promptly and less vigorously, and may require a repetition of the dose of tuberculin. Tuberculous infection of these nodes, which is active and producing pressure symptoms, may respond with a focal reaction characterized by an exaggeration of these symptoms. In cases with toxic symptoms, but no pressure symptoms, the latter may appear temporarily as the result of a focal reaction. With the subsidence of the reaction an improvement is seen, and not infrequently have I noted reactions, provoked for the purpose of confirming a diagnosis, prove to be the turning point in the course of the disease with marked improvement and even apparent recovery following. For these reasons I do not hesitate to employ the subcutaneous test as a means of diagnosis and when used, as I have directed, it can result in no harm and often has a most beneficial effect.

Complement Fixation Test.—The complement fixation test which has proven to be of so much value in the diagnosis and control of treatment in syphilis, has, in recent years, been applied along similar lines in the diagnosis of tuberculosis. The results reported thus far are somewhat conflicting and more work is needed, both in the laboratory and in clinical application of the test, before it can be placed upon a thoroughly practical basis and generally accepted as a routine diagnostic measure. The conflicting statements regarding the test are evidently due, in large part, to the fact that various workers with the test make use of different antigens.

Value of Different Antigens.—BESREDKA [13] using an antigen prepared from culture grown in egg bouillon obtains about 90% of positive results, being definite cases of tuberculosis, but the value of these observations is impaired by the fact that syphilitic cases would also give positive results. McINTOSH and FILDES [14] use as an antigen a freshly prepared emulsion of the bacilli in saline; they grow the bacilli used in preparing their antigen on glycerin egg medium. They quote the following results:

	Cases	Positive	Percentage
Phthisis	43	33	76.7
Surgical tuberculosis exclusive of glands	26	21	80.7
Tuberculous Glands	16	6	37.5

Eighty-seven control cases, taken from a variety of disease conditions in addition to normal individuals, were negative with the exception of three. Two of these were cases of leprosy in which the reaction may be explained as a "Group reaction."

The other was a case of Addison's disease in which tuberculosis is a frequent etiological factor. They tested the sera of eighteen syphilitics with positive Wasserman tests and all gave a negative reaction. With tuberculin as an antigen syphilitics frequently react. They conclude that the lesion must be of considerable size and constitute disease before it will give a reaction. "We look upon the positive reaction therefore as indicating positive tuberculosis." If such proves to be the case the complement fixation test will be of great value in diagnosis.

BRONFENBRENNER [15] uses Besredka's antigen. He concludes that the reaction is not lipotropic in nature. "When the serum deviates the complement in the presence of both Besredka's antigen and pure lipoid antigen, each of the two antigens can be exhausted from the serum independently of the other." He finds that the antigen does not lose its antigenic properties when freed of its lipoid substances. The evidence he brings forth points to the evident specificity of the test. He obtained 93.84% of positive reactions in active tuberculosis.

Craig's Polyvalent Antigen.—CRAIG [16] uses a polyvalent antigen prepared from several strains of bacilli. He finds complement binding bodies present in blood serum of individuals with either clinically active or inactive tuberculosis. He obtained positive reactions in 96.2% of cases of active and 66.1% of inactive tuberculosis. He found the test negative in normal individuals and not positive in syphilitics, if no tuberculosis was present. He concludes that, when positive, it is specific.

The complement fixation test may be negative in advanced cases of tuberculosis. Tuberculin tests are also often observed to be negative, in such cases indicating the absence of immune bodies from the serum of individuals so afflicted. The reaction may also be positive for some time after a lesion has become quiescent and inactive, as determined by the history and symptomatology.

Considering the limited amount of work, which has been done in this test, it is promising and deserves further study and trial.

The Agglutination Test.—ARLOING employed the agglutination method, based on the GRUBER-WIDAL reaction as used in typhoid, for the diagnosis of tuberculosis. In the case of tubercle bacilli it is difficult to make sure of agglutination. They grow slowly, and spontaneously occur in groups. Such cultures cannot be used in determining whether or not agglutination has occurred. In the test cultures, known as homogeneous cultures obtained by special technique, are employed. In such cultures the bacilli lie singly and are capable of agglutination or, more properly speaking, precipitation. The method has been employed by Arloing and others, the course of procedure is too complicated for ordinary use, the results are not sufficiently reliable for practical purposes, and the method is little used at present.

KINGHORN and TWITCHELL [17] found that the blood serum of healthy individuals agglutinated the tubercle bacilli almost as frequently as did the serum of patients suffering from pulmonary tuberculosis. They noted agglutination in 84.28% of healthy, as compared with 87.09% of tuberculous individuals.

Various other tests have been proposed from time to time but they have proven to be of little value in diagnosis. Wright's opsonic index is of no practical value. Arneth's blood picture was never advanced as a diagnostic method, but only as an aid in prognosis.

CHAPTER IX

TREATMENT

Prophylaxis.—In dealing with the treatment of any disease our first aim should be prophylaxis and prevention. Especially is this to be desired in a disease so prevalent and claiming so many victims as does tuberculosis, the treatment of which is tedious and often unsatisfactory. Prophylactic measures have proven inefficient in the past and are in need of revision. The measures employed should vary with the object aimed at, as the prevention of infection and the protection of adults and children differ.

The prevention of infection in infancy demands our first attention. Children are born free from tuberculosis, congenital infection being very rare, even if the parents were tuberculous at the time of conception and birth of the child. But many infants are infected during the first year of life and with increasing age the number increases, as can be demonstrated by the reaction to tuberculin, until at the age of 14 years, over 90% of all individuals have had a tuberculous infection. Tuberculosis is a very dangerous disease in infants who exhibit but little resistance to it. During the first two years of life infection is likely to result in an acute or subacute disease which proves fatal in nearly all cases. After infancy it becomes less dangerous and less often causes death although it may localize in the glands or bones and cause a prolonged period of ill health and perhaps disfigurement. In combating infantile tuberculosis we should aim at the prevention of infection and at the increase of the powers of resistance of the body. Because of the fatality of infantile tuberculosis, it is clear that our aim should be to protect infants under two years of age from infection, and to subject older children to the contagion of the tubercle bacillus as rarely and as late in life as possible. This is a simple matter in families, in which there is no tuberculous member, but a difficult problem presents itself, when the child is exposed to infection by contact with members of his own immediate family, who are suffering from the disease.

Children Must be Removed from the Infected.—No infant should be allowed to remain in a home with an individual suffering from phthisis. Either the infected individual or the infant must be removed. Even consumptives, who are cleanly, and are careful about the disposal of their sputum, and of little or no danger to adults, are dangerous to the susceptible infant. Special difficulties are encountered when one of the parents has tuberculosis. The tuberculous individual who marries and has a family takes upon himself a great responsibility. Individuals, whose tuberculosis is not positively healed, should be encouraged not to marry. If they do so they should be informed of the dangers their children would be subjected to, and procreation should not be permitted, unless they are willing to have their children removed from them for two years after birth, a wish rarely complied with. From animal experiments we may infer that children so cared for will be healthy. Hess [1] has called attention to the neglect to provide for the welfare of the infants born of tuberculous parentage and urges that, in the light of our present knowledge as to the time when infection occurs and the fatality of infantile tuberculosis, our methods of prophylaxis be reconstructed. No tuberculous mother should be allowed to rear her children at least during infancy, for very few survive when nursed by such a mother. After delivery the child should be removed to surroundings, where it will not be subjected to the dangers of infection, and should not be permitted in the proximity of the tuberculous mother for the first two years of life. Hess advised the establishment of preventoriums for infants where they should receive adequate care. It is rarely that such radical wishes are complied with, for mothers will not part with their children, unless they are in the last stages of the disease. Many such mothers have the care of their household and cannot be spared. Likewise, the tuberculous father may be a menace but cannot be spared and removed to a sanitorium, for he may be the only source of income. If the infant cannot be removed from the house, the most painstaking precautions must be observed and, so far as possible, it should be isolated from the infected individual. Whenever possible the care of the infant should be entrusted to a healthy individual and when a tuberculous mother is compelled, by necessity, to assume the personal care of the infant she should be fully instructed as to the dangers of the infection and the means to be adopted for preventing them. In houses where there is no tuberculous individual the protection of the infant is an easier matter. Strangers should be forbidden to fondle children, and the kissing of infants is particularly objectionable.

Nurses and Servants Should be Examined.—In selecting a nurse or servant who comes into intimate association, tuberculosis should be thought of and anyone suffering from open tuberculosis should not be permitted to mingle with children.

Resistance.—In addition the general precautions for increasing the powers of resistance of the body should be observed. The question of feeding is of prime importance and whenever possible infants should be breast fed, for such children have greater resistance against all infections, including tuberculosis. Only in the most incipient stages should a tuberculous mother be allowed to nurse her child for the number infected by contact with mothers suffering from open tuberculosis is very great. The danger is in contact, and not in the transmission of infection by the milk. Mother's milk is the ideal and safest food for the infant. A wet nurse is the next choice, but is seldom available, and it then becomes necessary to resort to artificial feeding as a substitute. One should endeavor for the first few weeks, the most serious time, to obtain nourishment for the child from the mother and then should a change be necessary cow's milk properly modified may be substituted, at first for only one meal, and then two or three or more may be given, but breast milk should always be given as long as possible, at least during the first six months of life.

Milk an Important Factor.—When artificial feeding becomes necessary the dangers of bovine infection must be thought of. Milk for infant feeding should be obtained from cattle, free from tuberculosis as demonstrated by tuberculin tests, and obtained from dairies where the best of sanitary conditions prevail. In cities such milk is obtainable in the form of certified milk, the only drawback of which is its rather high cost. Raw milk is, in many ways, preferable, but when the source of supply is unknown and the methods of handling and delivery are not beyond suspicion some method of sterilization is imperative. Pasteurization is the most satisfactory method and presents the least objections. Intense heating of the milk is undesirable although boiling is more certain. However, tubercle bacilli are killed by an exposure of 140° F. maintained for 20 minutes, and this temperature does not render the milk unfit for use, or impair its nutritive properties.

Fresh Air.—Tuberculosis is a house disease and care should be exercised in the home to which children are more or less closely confined for the first years of their life. Fresh air, light, and cleanliness are cardinal demands to which attention should be paid for hygienic reasons. Fresh air has an invigorating influence upon the nourishment of any individual. Air within homes is never so pure or free from germs as the open air and children should, therefore, be accustomed to fresh air at an early age, avoiding, of course, needless exposures and radical attempts at hardening. Sunlight and fresh air are the enemies of the tubercle bacillus, and homes should be lighted and well ventilated, especially the nursery. A light airy home is a more important factor in the life of the child than of the adult, whose activities take him into the open air to a greater extent.

Cleanliness.—Children and their environments should be kept clean. Rooms in which children live should be cleansed daily and aired several times a day, for frequent sunning and ventilation will help to exterminate any tubercle bacilli that may be present. People in changing residence from one place to another should always consieer the possibility of their predecessors having had tuberculosis, and should cleanse and disinfect accordingly. Children old enough to creep are especially liable to become infected from contaminated carpets and floors. Hence, carpets should be banished whenever possible and replaced by rugs, which can more easily be removed and thoroughly cleansed.

The floors should be kept clean and not trodden upon with dirty shoes, as creeping children, if allowed their freedom, come in constant contact with them. It is a good plan to confine children of this age in one part of the room upon a clean sheet. Dry sweeping and dusting are to be avoided because of the dangers of dust infection.

The improved method of vacuum cleansing is an advancement and, when not available, cleansing of the floors and removal of dust should be accomplished by a damp cloth. The child's toys should be washable and frequently cleansed.

Dangers From Outside Infection.—In older children the contact with individuals, outside the immediate family, makes the prevention of all infection difficult. But the contact is less intimate and the infection less massive and goes on to healing, or becomes a latent glandular infection which becomes serious only under special circumstances. The mortality of tuberculosis in older children is slight and in striking contrast to that in infancy. These mild infections act as a vaccination against tuberculosis, and upon this probably depends the protection of the race from the ravages of tuberculosis. Our object then should be to prevent all infection during infancy and to prevent massive infection of older children.

Our attempts at protection from tuberculosis in older children should not be so much directed against the prevention of infection, which is almost inevitably acquired, as toward protecting them from the consequences of what has already occurred and cannot be avoided. The comparative harmlessness of these infections is evidenced by the fact that almost everyone has had some tuberculous infection, and yet only a certain percentage die of tuberculosis. A dangerous feature lies in the fact that the transition of a harmless latent infection to tuberculous disease is so gradual that it is usually overlooked, until disaster has resulted.

Important to Examine all Children.—In order to recognize the existence of tuberculous disease in its incipiency, MARY E. LAPHAM [2] recommends the medical examination of school children. She states that: "The competent yearly examination of every child in the public schools, if not ruined by political appointments, will detect the beginnings of tuberculous processes, where and when they start in children, and eventually teach us that the danger from the tubercle bacillus is far more from within than from without. Infection does not always cause tuberculosis, but if it should, then the sooner we find it out the better."

Glandular Infections.—In preventing glandular tuberculosis we must direct attention to the mucous membranes of the respiratory and gastro-intestinal tracts, which are tributary to the commonly affected bronchial, cervical and mesenteric glands. In the gastro-intestinal tract, we should avoid digestive disturbances and inflammations. Although the tubercle bacillus can pass through a healthy mucous membrane and infect the adjacent glands, the chances of infection are greatly increased in the presence of an inflammation. In this regard, overfeeding of infants with cows' milk is more to be feared than underfeeding. The excess of food passes through the intestinal tract undigested and non-used. Continuous over feeding may irritate the mucous membrane by the process of decomposition, and lead to inflammation and swelling of the lymphatic follicles, which favors gland infection and lessens absorption and impairs nutrition. It goes without saying, that we must quickly relieve underfeeding both quantitative and qualitative. A form of qualitative underfeeding observed in older children is fat starvation. Many children presenting themselves for treatment of glandular tuberculosis give a history of marked aversion to fats. This should be combated, for fats are essential to good nutrition.

Respiratory Tract a Source of Danger.—Attention must be paid to the respiratory tract with the view of preventing reinfection from within the body. Latent infections may lie dormant in the bronchial glands and only become active under special circumstances. Impaired nutrition and lowered resistance, incident to intercurrent disease, seem to be the most potent factors in activating such infections and causing tuberculous disease. Young children and infants are to be protected from measles, pertussis, scarlet fever, and other infectious diseases, during which an allergic state is known to occur. It seems that the younger the child the more is the allergy induced likely to be followed by active tuberculosis. Special care is to be taken in case of children of tuberculous parentage, for they have probably been subjected to a massive infection. If these infectious diseases do occur, children should be guarded against them until four or five years of age. Attention must be given such children during convalescence, with a view of increasing their bodily resistance, by giving proper and adequate nourishment, and securing an out-door life.

Diseased Tonsils Must be Removed.—We should watch for and correct any physical abnormalities that may be present. Obstructions to breathing particularly demand early attention. Diseased tonsils and adenoids are common portals of entry of the tubercle bacillus in infections of the cervical nodes. Removal of such diseased tissues is always indicated because of the obstruction to breathing and dangers of infection, and is very frequently followed by subsidence of glandular swellings, but there is little reason to believe that even a complete removal will do more than slightly aid in the cure, if the tubercle bacilli have passed from the tonsils or adenoids to the nodes. A tonsillectomy sometimes immediately accelerates the tuberculous disease in the nodes. Such operation, however, is an adjuvant to direct treatment, and is to be considered in every case. If tonsils are not inflamed, or are not hypertrophic and obstructive, it is wiser not to remove them for no indication for such a measure then exists. By removing healthy tonsils we are producing an interruption of the tonsillar ring of Waldeyer, and may we not in so doing lower the resistance of those structures to the advent of infection?

General Treatment.—The general treatment of glandular tuberculosis must be supportive and symptomatic. Supportive treatment relates mainly to the hygiene of living and to the diet. Ocean and mountain climates are to be considered and when desirable and possible, a change in climate is indicated. Fresh air is essential and whenever possible the patient should be in the fresh air day and night. A proper amount of rest is essential, even when there is no fever or other signs of toxæmia present. When the temperature goes above 99.5° F. or other definite toxic signs present themselves, absolute rest is imperative. Patients that are about should take a definite amount of rest during the day and plenty of sleep at night.

Dietetic Treatment.—Proper dietetics are important in the treatment of any form of tuberculosis, under the influence of which the subcutaneous and other deposits of fat disappear, and the muscles decrease in size and in tone. To counteract this tendency and to supply energy for the needs of the body in maintaining its equilibrium and combating the tuberculous disease, food of proper quantity and quality is essential. All individuals thrive best on a mixed diet. The food should be nutritious and energy producing and rather rich in fats. The amount of food given will depend upon the requirements of the individual patient. The most reliable guide to a patient's condition is his gain in weight, and he should therefore be weighed weekly, and his food consumption regulated accordingly. Not only must the food be given in relative abundance, but it must possess quality and variety and be supplied in goodly amount. Fat is essential to the tuberculous individual in maintaining his nutrition and aiding him in the combat with his disease. That tuberculous individuals often show a marked aversion for fats is a common observation. Fat is best supplied in the form of rich milk, cream and butter. These foods are quite rich in fat and are easily obtainable, being articles of ordinary diet, and palatable. Fresh pure milk, or some of its many modifications are of great value, and should be given in quantities of one or two quarts daily. Milk, diluted with vichy or carbonated water, can be tolerated when plain milk ofttimes cannot.

The value of fat in the treatment of tuberculosis was recognized in the use of cod liver oil. Although formerly considered as a medicinal agent, and its therapeutic value attributed to substances such as iodides contained in it in traces, its value must be conceded to be due to its fat content, and it may properly be classed among the food stuffs. On account of its fatty acid content it is easily digested and assimilated. It is employed preferably for thin excitable children. The lighter clear refined oils are preferable, being milder and less unpleasant to take. Many children will take the oil pure, while for others the taste must be disguised. It may be given in the form of an emulsion, or in combination with malt. It should be given after meals and given over a long period of time, since it possesses food value only. It can be given for months in the winter time, but it may be necessary to interrupt it in the summer or at any time if it causes digestive disturbances, such as eructations, anorexia, nausea, vomiting or diarrhœa. Its use should not be insisted upon if there is great dislike for it.

Many foods are available. In nutritive value and in ease of assimilation, eggs are second only to milk and are subject to a variety of preparation. Meats should be given in moderation, and the more robust may take many kinds variously prepared. Fried meats are harder to digest. Carbohydrate food is available in many forms. Alcohol is contraindicated.

Dangers in Overfeeding.—The food stuffs prescribed for any patient should be adapted to the digestive powers and tastes of that individual patient. Overfeeding is to be avoided for it is harmful. A patient is overfed when he takes and absorbs more than is required for his energy exchanges. The important point is, not what a tuberculous patient eats but what he can digest and assimilate. An excess of food not digested and absorbed is likely to cause alimentary disturbances. A too great increase in weight due to the deposition of fat is inadvisable, for fat is relatively inactive and an excess adds little to one's powers of resistance.

Tuberculin Treatment.—The use of tuberculin in treatment of tuberculosis was first introduced by Koch, a few years after his discovery of the tubercule bacillus. The great hopes that were placed on tuberculin at first were soon shattered The enormous doses administered, instead of curing the disease, resulted often in marked aggravation of the symptoms and apparently, in many cases, hastened the end.

Due to these unfortunate experiences, tuberculin came into disfavor amongst the medical profession at large and would

certainly have lost its place entirely in the treatment of tuberculosis, if not a few men had seen the real cause for its apparent
failure.

The administration of large doses was discontinued by these
men and replaced by minute doses. Due to the excellent work
done by these investigators, especially in Germany, the interest
in tuberculin was again aroused and further investigations have
fully proven to men of unbiased minds that tuberculin has a
distinct place in the treatment of tuberculosis.

No Substitute Offered by the Men who Condemn Tuberculin.— .
In America tuberculin has never had a universal use. A few
men, however, have clung to it steadily during the time of its
evolution. Tuberculin has often been condemned by the profession at large. But a change in opinion is bound to come, the
work of many men in our country, giving absolute proof of the
value of tuberculin, will without question, in due time, get the
recognition it deserves.

Tuberculin of to-day is not the last word in treatment of tuberculosis; far be it from me to assume it. But of all the remedies
that have been projected tuberculin, in my opinion, stands so
much in advance of any other single agent that it cannot be
thrown aside by the conscientious practitioner.

Varieties of Tuberculin.—A large number of tuberculins have
been discovered both for diagnostic and therapeautic purposes,
Many of our foremost authors on the subject of tuberculosis.
notably WOLFF-EISNER and SAHLI, consider that the active
principle in all the tuberculins is very much the same, being a
tuberculo-protein. This is, according to SAHLI,[3] proven by the
exactly similar character of the so-called tuberculin reactions
which can be produced by all tuberculins without exception.
But we know that variations as to degree of reaction are manifested by the various preparations. This is undoubtedly due
to the differences in the constituent portions of the various
tuberculin-proteins, fats and toxins being present in different
amounts and different degrees of availability.[4]

Koch's Old Tuberculin.—The original article discovered by
KOCH and called "Koch's Old Tuberculin," has served as a

basis for nearly all new varieties and is considered by many as the tuberculin par excellence. It is made by growing a culture in a glycerinated (5%) alkaline broth for six to eight weeks, which is then sterilized and concentrated to one-tenth of its original volume and finally filtered through a Berkefeld filter. Old tuberculin, therefore, is a glycerinated extract of the bacillary bodies, containing also the products which were formed during their growth, and also some extraneous material from the culture medium. The peptone contents of the latter, although very minute in quantity, caused Koch to manufacture his albumose-free tuberculin, which is identical with the old with the exception that it is grown on asparagin culture medium and hence does not contain any peptone bodies.

Other varieties are Koch's new tuberculin (T. R.) which at present is hardly used at all. Koch's bacillary emulsion, by many considered the most valuable of all tuberculins, scarcely contains anything else than the most finely powdered body-substance of the tubercle bacilli. The sensitized bacillary emulsion of MEYERS, which, in addition to bacillary bodies, also contains tuberculous serum. BERANECK's tuberculin, strongly recommended by SAHLI, is grown on peptone-free culture media and is essentially a mixture of tubercle broth, filtered free from bacilli and evaporated down to vacuo at a low temperature, with an extract of the bodies of tubercle bacilli made with orthophosphoric acid. This latter, therefore, contains the bacillary protein in the form of an acid orthophosphate of albumin.

Constituents of Tuberculin.—The more recent investigations, into the question of tuberculin, show a distinct tendency to separate the bacillary bodies into their simpler compounds, proteins, fats, etc. VAUGHN has separated one soluble and one insoluble protein; DEYCKE and MUCH have produced various partial antigens belonging to the protein, fat and toxin groups; v. RUCK has isolated several proteins. POTTENGER [5] is undoubtedly right in assuming that the work of these men is pointing the way to future improvements in the production of specific tubercle vaccines.

Action of Tuberculin.—The specific action of tuberculin is that of active immunization, hence a few words about the subject of immunity with regard to tuberculosis are not amiss.

Immunity to tuberculosis is a very much disputed question at the present time. The opinions vary from one extreme to the other. Some observers do not believe that any immunity exists whatsoever against this dreadful disease. Others believe that it is immunity which plays the foremost rôle in saving the human race from complete extinction.

Natural immunity is the resistance to infection, normally possessed, usually as the result of inheritance, by certain individuals or species under natural conditions. The existence of this form of immunity is very hard to prove. REIBMAYR [6] believes that he has proved it for single families who, in the struggle for life, have acquired and handed down from generation to generation a resistance to tuberculosis by having recovered from the disease.

An apparent support of this is the severe nature of the disease when it attacks races of people who have not before been in contact with tuberculosis. For instance, the negroes in Africa are very susceptible to the disease and the fatality is enormous. The American Indian fell an easy prey to the White Man's Great White Plague; more recently has DEYCKE [7] reported the condition amongst Turks who, it appears, have not come into contact with tuberculosis to a marked extent until recently. Amongst them the disease shows itself in a very acute and severe form and has a malignant course.

The contention then seems reasonable that amongst those living in contact with tuberculosis there must be a very real, if only a relative immunity. To express it in BULLOCK's words [8]— "Physicians or no physicians, science or no science, nature is quietly, but none the less persistently and effectively, immunizing the human race against tuberculosis." An analogy may here be seen with what has occurred in lues and leprosy.

But the question has arisen if this severe form of tuberculosis attacking new races is not caused by the absence of the protective influence of a mild infection during childhood.

The question of ACQUIRED IMMUNITY thus arises. It has often

been said that the difference in reaction to tuberculosis in children and adults is due to the difference in age. In view of the
recent investigations this supposition does not seem to hold true.
The individual reacts in one way to the original infection, may
it occur in childhood or adult life; in another way to super or
reinfection. Hence, the similarity between the disease of childhood, when a severe infection is present, and that of adults in a
race recently exposed to the disease.

KOCH's phenomenon, without question, constitutes the most
important research in immunity to tuberculosis. His experiments
are so classical and their importance so great that a detailed
description is not malplaced.[9]

"When one vaccinates a healthy guinea-pig with a pure culture of
tubercle bacilli, the wound, as a rule, closes and in the first few days
seems to heal. However, in from ten to fourteen days a hard nodule
appears which soon breaks down, leaving an ulcer that persists to the
time of death of the animal. There is quite a different sequence of
events when a tuberculous guinea-pig is vaccinated; for this, animals
are best suited that have been successfully infected for four to six weeks
previously. In such an animal the inoculation would also promptly
unite. However, no nodule forms, but on the next or second day after
a peculiar change occurs. The point of inoculation and the tissues
about, over an area of 0.1 to 1 c.m. in diameter grow hard and take on
a dark discoloration. Observation on subsequent days makes it more
and more apparent that the altered skin is necrotic. It is finally cast
off and a shallow ulceration remains which usually heals quickly and
permanently without the neighbouring lymph-glands becoming infected. Inoculated tubercle bacilli act very differently upon the
skin of healthy and tuberculous guinea-pigs. This striking action is
not restricted to living tubercle bacilli, but is equally manifested by
dead bacilli whether they be killed by exposure to low temperature,
for a long time, or to the boiling temperature, or by the action of various chemicals.

"After having discovered these remarkable facts I followed them up
in all directions and was further able to show that killed pure cultures
of tubercle bacilli, ground up and suspended in water, can be injected
in large amounts under the skin of healthy guinea-pigs without producing any other effect than local suppuration. Tuberculous guinea-

pigs, on the other hand, are killed in from six to forty-eight hours, according to the dose given, by the injection of small quantities of such suspension. A dose which just falls short of the amount necessary to kill the animal may produce extensive necrosis of the skin about the point of injection. If the suspension be diluted until it is just visibly cloudy, the injected animals remain alive, and if the administration is continued with one or two intervals, a rapid improvement in their condition takes place; the ulcerating inoculation wound becomes smaller, and is finally replaced by a scar, a process that never takes place without such treatment; the swollen lymph-glands become smaller, the nutrition improves and the disease process, unless it is too far advanced and the animals die of exhaustion, comes to a standstill."

ROMER, one of our foremost students on immunity in tuberculosis, has substantiated the findings of KOCH and has also, in a most striking manner, proved that protective vaccination is possible in cattle and sheep. He vaccinated cattle with living tubercle bacilli of a human strain, non-lethal for cattle.[10] When these animals were later subjected to the inoculation of a large dose of virulent tubercle bacilli they showed an immediate reaction of rise in temperature. But this gradually subsided and a complete cure resulted. The controls of non-vaccinated animals, however, reacted in the usual manner and soon died from typical inoculation tuberculosis. ROMER vaccinated sheep in the same manner, using bovine tubercle bacilli.[11] Sheep, according to this investigator, approach men in their resistance to tuberculous infection. A sheep infected subcutaneously August 6, 1908, with virulent bovine tubercle bacilli, and reinfected intravenously with more than double the number of the same bacilli on March 3, 1909, when killed September 1, 1909, showed but trifling tuberculous changes, those that were present being similar to and not of greater extent than those found in a control animal which had received the first, but not the second injection, while the control of the second injection died in two months with enormous tuberculosis of the lungs.

In his experiments on guinea-pigs, ROMER showed that the immunity enjoyed after reinfection was not due to the fact that the tubercle bacilli had all been destroyed, for a bit of apparently unaltered skin over the site of reinfection in the tuberculous guinea-pig being cut out and injected in a free guinea-pig caused the death of the animal from typical inoculation tuberculosis.

Bearing these investigations in mind, when considering the question of tuberculosis in men, some conclusions seem justified. BULLOCK [12] remarks that the lifelong and very practical immunity possessed by the six-sevenths of the human family must be largely the result of a primary and insignificant infection with its resulting sensitization, or, as might be said, state of preparedness.

If we consider the enormous number of adults who react to tuberculin, without having any clinical manifestations of tuberculosis whatsoever, we must conclude that a positive v. Pirquet tuberculin reaction is not a sign of active disease, but only shows that the individual has had a tuberculous infection. Hence, all cases of tuberculosis are not progressive; some cases may be cured, and some have, as MUCH [13] says, acquired a certain degree of immunity, overcoming the initial infection as is shown by the presence of a large amount of immune bodies. MUCH further argues that the constant exposure of man to tuberculosis, without question, causes repeated infections but that the individual, by virtue of his acquired immunity, easily conquers them. On account of these repeated attacks are the body defenses strengthened, and the immune bodies increased in number. This may give an explanation for the presence of antibodies in the individual, years after the initial infection in childhood.

In view of these arguments the truth in LOWENSTEIN's ambiguous statement is clearly seen—"Only the tuberculous are tuberculosis immune." The calcified bronchial glands have been called the vaccination mark of tuberculosis. In truth, a proper name. But for this protection, acquired of course at great risk to the child, it is presumed by some that adult human beings would be as susceptible to first infections as adults of other animals are known to be. As F. C. SMITH [14] says, "the immunity of adults is, therefore, no great cause for congratulation; it is attained at too great a price."

Theories of Reaction to Tuberculin.—Healthy animals do not react to tuberculin when the latter is injected in moderate doses.

In tuberculous animals, on the other hand, the injection of the most minute amounts cause a profound change in the body-equilibrium; the temperature is raised, signs of marked activity appear at the seat of disease and some changes at the site of administration of the tuberculin. The manifestations of the reaction have been fully discussed in the chapter on Tuberculin Diagnosis.

Many theories have been proposed to explain the phenomena of tuberculin reactions. The first suggestion was that tuberculin acts so powerfully in an infected individual by reason of the fact that a certain amount of it is present in the organism, having been formed in the tuberculous focus. The addition of injected tuberculin to that already present in the circulation causes the general reaction, and its addition to that in the focus causes the focal reaction. This summation theory, in many respects, fails to offer a complete or satisfactory explanation and may, therefore, be discarded.

Wasserman and Bruck's Theory.—A more recent theory is that of WASSERMAN and BRUCK.[15] Following the success of the complement deviation reaction in the diagnosis and control of treatment in syphilis they applied the reaction to the study of serum of tuberculous individuals. They found an immune body, or amboceptor, which they term "anti-tuberculin" and which, with tuberculin, binds complement. Upon this basis they attempted to explain the tuberculin reactions, believing the complement fixation to be the cause. They conclude that a focal reaction occurs after the injection of tuberculin, the antituberculin meeting the antigen tuberculin and fixing complement in the tuberculous focus. This causes the softening of the tissues of the focus and the focal reaction, the protein digesting power being attributed to the fixed complement. The general and febrile reactions are due to the absorption of products from the softened tubercular tissue. The general reaction is thus made secondary to the focal reaction. The theory has not given an entirely satisfactory explanation of the tuberculin reaction, but has excited interest and stimulated research work in complement deviation in tuberculosis.

Sahli's Objection.—SAHLI [16] calls attention to objections to the theory. He considers it "quite incomprehensible how tuberculin and antituberculin can exist simultaneously in tuberculous foci without neutralizing one another under the influence of complement which is always present." He also finds the explanation of inflammatory reactions unsatisfactory since the chemical affinities are satisfied, and considers that the action of complement would be directed to the combination of tuberculin and antituberculin rather than to digestion of the tissues.

v. Pirquet and Schick's Views.—v. PIRQUET [17] observed that an organism which has gone through an infection changes its power of reaction to the same causative agent; this change, the so-called allergic reaction, is seen most clearly when an extract of the infective agent is inoculated into the skin. He and SCHICK held that the tuberculin reaction is due to the formation of toxic substances as a result of the combination of antibodies and the injected tuberculin. This formation of toxin may occur locally and in the blood-stream as well, thus accounting for both the local and general reactions.

Wolff-Eisner's Theory.—WOLFF-EISNER [18] has modified the theory of WASSERMAN and BRUCK. He observed that "the first injection of a foreign albuminous substance produces no immunity but always hypersensitiveness which is evident on the second injection of the same albuminous substance." He believes in the existence in tuberculosis of an antibody of the nature of an amboceptor, which according to him, is lytic in character. He concludes that specific lysins are elaborated by the organism, which are able to break up complex molecular aggregates, setting free from the foreign proteins by this lytic action, endotoxin-like substances which exhibit an increased toxic action. He assumes that the active principle in the tuberculin consists of ultra-microscopic fragments of the bacteria, hence a foreign albuminous material which is of comparatively low toxicity as evidenced by the large doses tolerated by those who are free from tuberculous infection. The sensitive tuberculous person has this specific lysin in his body as the result of his infection, and the antibody, the bacteriolytic amboceptor, under the action of complement unlocks, so to speak, or splits the tuberculo-protein into secondary products, less complex molecules of high toxicity, which have an irritative action on the tuberculous foci, thus producing the focal reaction. The general reaction occurring simultaneously is due to the action of these same toxins on the system in general. This presupposes then that the tuberculin which has become lysinized and being, therefore, toxic is neutralized by the protective reaction of the organism by the formation of antitoxic antibodies.

Theory of Anaphylaxis.—The modern tendency is to consider the tuberculin reaction as an allergic or anaphylactic reaction phenomenon. Early observations of anaphylactic reactions were made by PORTRER, ARTHUS, THEOBALD SMITH and others when they demonstrated that sensitization to serums and toxins was manifested by a severe reaction when a second injection was given after an interval of several days had elapsed. Such substances have received the name of anaphylactogens since they produce a specific hypersusceptibility after an incubation period of at least five to seven days.

Anaphylactogens are proteins or are inseparably connected with proteins. The parenteral introduction of an anaphylactogen leads to the production of a specific antibody termed anaphylactin. Several days are required for the production of this antibody, or immune substance, thus accounting for the incubation period. The subsequent injection of anaphylactogen leads to the reaction. VAUGHN and others consider that the process of sensitization consists in the development of specific proteolytic ferments, and the reaction to enzymatic proteolysis by means of which the foreign protein is broken up into toxic substances.

Vaughn's Theory.—VAUGHN [19] has shown that proteins can be hydralized with alcohol and sodium hydrate into one portion with highly toxic action and another portion which showed marked sensitizing property but little toxicity. These principles of anaphylaxis can easily be applied to the explanation of the tuberculin reaction. The tuberculin formed in the tuberculous focus leads to the production of specific proteolytic ferments and the organism is thus sensitized. When tuberculin is introduced from without the ferments act upon it and liberate the toxic element; the reactions result from its irritant action upon the body cells. The similarity of this theory and WOLFF-EISNER'S is readily seen; he speaks of a lytic amboceptor, and VAUGHN, and others, adherents of the anaphylaxis theory, of proteolytic ferment.

While the fundamental hypothesis of the theory of parenteral digestion, as developed by VAUGHN and others, has been generally accepted, there is some difference of opinion as to the mechanism by which it is formed in the body. According to the early assumption, it is entirely an intra-vascular affair; this is substantiated by the experiments of BIEDL and KRAUS, FRIEDEMANN and others,[20] which shows that all the factors necessary for the production of allergic reactions may be present in the blood-stream. Recent researches, however, seem to place marked importance upon cellular reactivity. PEARCE and EISENBERG [21] using transfusion methods, SCHULTZ, DALE and WEIL [22] using isolated muscle tissue of sensitized animals, have shown conclusively that the conditions of hypersensitiveness is largely determined by an increased capacity for reaction on the part of the fixed cells to the specific antigen, probably occasioned by an excess of specific antibodies or enzymes in the protoplasm.

General Action.—Tuberculin treatment consists essentially of an immunizing healing action which is not, however, a complete immunization but only a relative one. This relative immunity presupposes an increase in the capacity for resistance by the stimulation of all the anatomical and physiological processes which are so frequently causative in the spontaneous healing of tuberculous lesions.

The process of immunization consists of raising the natural capacity present in the organism of reacting to the tuberculous toxin. In tuberculin immunization the body primarily tolerates increasing quantities of tuberculin, but also renders inocuous the toxins elaborated in the tuberculous foci.

Whether or not the tuberculin contains the real toxin of tubercle bacilli is still not determined. Those who have assumed the negative, base their opinion largely upon the fact that complete immunization to tuberculosis by means of tuberculin cannot be obtained. The production of tubercles by tuberculin apparently leaves but little doubt that the same toxin is found both in tuberculin and tubercle bacilli. SAHLI basing his opinion upon the lysin theory, concludes that the difference in action between the tubercle bacilli and tuberculin is merely one of degree.

The v. RUCKS are of the opinion that actively acquired immunity against bacillus tuberculosis is not produced against its secretions and body constituents simultaneously. They maintain that this immunity is established gradually. First, against the toxins elaborated by the living tubercle bacilli, and later against the constituents of the bacillus in direct proportion to their solubility and rapidity of destruction of the bacillus. This is necessarily slow because the bacillus is resistent to solvents and also are enclosed in non-vascular tubercles.

The specific actions of the substances which are concerned in production of immunity, such as antitoxins, agglutinins, precipitins, aggressins, opsosins, etc., can be studied in modern works on immunity.

Local Action.—The local action of tuberculin upon the focus of infection is one of the greatest importance, and is undoubtedly dependent upon the inflammatory hyperemia produced. This increases the phagocytic activity of the leucocytes which, though present in the natural course of tuberculosis, are increased by tuberculin treatment. Through this local hyperemia actual healing of lesion is produced with absorption of the diseased tissue and formation of new connective tissue.

Indications for the Use of Tuberculin.—The use of tuberculin in treatment of tuberculosis of the lymphatic system has, in my experience, produced very fortunate results.

Tuberculous adenitis in any stage lends itself with great hope of success to the treatment with tuberculin; cases with suppurating glands are markedly improved and often subside without any surgical interference whatever. In some cases simple aspiration of glandular abscess seems necessary before healing can take place. Old cases of tuberculous adenitis with chronic discharging sinuses, which have been operated on time and time again without any apparent result, often yield to a long continued tuberculin treatment.

Contraindications to tuberculin, as it is administered at the present time, are few indeed. Advanced Bright's disease, decompensated heart lesions, pregnancy, acute infections, diabetes, and markedly advanced cases of pulmonary tuberculosis.

Method of Administrations.—In the discussion of the specific diagnosis of tuberculosis, I presented my views in regard to the dosage of tuberculin in the subcutaneous test, and emphasized that only comparatively small amounts of tuberculin were necessary to excite a reaction. The importance of this is paramount. The reaction to tuberculin, when it occurs, is an uncontrollable factor and may undoubtedly, in some cases, lead to unfavorable results—hence, the importance to select your cases.

Our strife in treatment of tuberculosis is to carry on the same without exciting any apparent reaction. In cases of glandular tuberculosis the danger is less than in pulmonary tuberculosis but should, however, be kept in mind. A reaction may indeed be of value in some cases and hasten recovery, acting as a marked stimulus to production of antibodies.

One should always remember, as BANDELIER and ROEPKE [23] have stated, that tuberculin does not contain any readymade healing factors, but they are produced by the organism itself as an anti-action against the poison.

The smallest dose of tuberculin undoubtedly is accompanied by some reactive changes, both generally and locally. The dose to do the most good would be one that produced the greatest amount of focal reaction without eliciting a general reaction, the latter as manifested by rise in temperature and other signs of toxic surcharge.

The irritative action upon the focal lesion produces tissue damage, associated with hyperæmia, and is the important factor in recovery, as long as it does not exceed the optimum amount of damage. When tissue damage is excessive, the progress of the disease is facilitated with the occurrence of favor and extension of inflammation in the tuberculous foci.

Toxic Phenomena, Indicative of a Reaction. The typical reac-

tions to a diagnostic dose of tuberculin have been discussed under
the subject of specific diagnosis and should always be avoided
during the progress of treatment. More subtle findings, however,
make their appearance when we are nearing the zone of danger.
During the progress of tuberculin treatment the patient should
show a distinct general improvement. The first signs to appear
in case patient is not reacting properly are often overlooked.
They may apparently be so insignificant as to be considered of
no value, but the physician should always be on the lookout.
The patient may begin to show symptoms of a general indisposi-
tion, become irritable, lose his appetite and consequently lose
weight. The latter is by many considered one of the most
valuable signs of trouble ahead. It is often the only finding,
indicative of lack of response. Hence, the marked importance
of weighing the patients at regular intervals to ascertain the
proper facts.

Acceleration of the pulse is emphasized by some authors as a
very important factor as indicative of untoward reaction. The
temperature, of course, plays an important rôle and is often the
only means whereby some clinicians control their doses. The
slightest rise in temperature should be looked at askance as a
possible forerunner of a marked reaction. The slightest rise
should have subsided before the next injection is given.

If any of the above signs of hypersensitiveness do appear,
the increase in dosage should be very gradual indeed. Oftentimes
it is imperative to repeat the same dose several times before
toximmunity for that particular dose is reached. In some cases
we find signs of accumulative action with a typical reaction following the repetition of the same dose. In these cases treatment
must be suspended for one to two weeks, and the next injection
must not be increased, and the subsequent increase in dosage must
be undertaken very carefully.

The way to administer tuberculin is by subcutaneous injection.
Other methods have been tried; orally, rectally by suppositories,
etc., but their failure has been demonstrated.

The site of injection varies with different men. Some prefer
the back, others the tissues of anterior aspect of the chest. Per-

sonally, I nearly always use the tissues of the arm. This area undoubtedly is somewhat more sensitive to local reaction than the others, and sometimes a local reaction may occur which, if of small volume, may be disregarded. This local affair undoubtedly is caused by the trace of tuberculin left in the skin during introduction of the needle, and hence may be regarded as a modified v. Pirquet reaction.

Time for Injection.—Tuberculin is usually administered in the morning when practicable. The reason for this is manifest. A reaction to tuberculin often occurs with 4-6 hours and in such a case a possible rise in temperature would be noted, whereas if administered in the afternoon or evening it would be overlooked during sleeping hours. Another reason is, that the usual afternoon rise of temperature is followed by the customary fall the following morning. If tuberculin is injected in the afternoon a febrile reaction, which may occur the following morning, may be obscured by the morning drop in temperature.

Dosage an Individual Question.—Tuberculin does not truly immunize the organism, but merely strives at increasing the capacity of the organism for anti-action. As this capacity for anti-action is different in each patient, the dosage varies accordingly and hence resolves itself into a study of each individual. The strength of the initial dose varies with the age of the patient, the presence or not of fever, of marked hypersensitiveness, etc. The initial dose should be repeated several times to demonstrate the presence or not of any cumulative action. If signs of this appear, the next dose should be withheld until they disappear.

The individuality of the treatment should never be lost sight of. We are dealing with a powerful therapeutic agent which has to be handled very carefully if we want to get the best results. The physician should always be on the lookout for signs of possible toxic reaction, the reactionless treatment being the ideal to obtain. The slightest toxic irritation signs absolutely indicate a prolongation of the intervals between injections.

In the treatment of glandular tuberculosis I use very small doses throughout the entire course of treatment—smaller than in pulmonary tuberculosis. This with clear understanding of the fact that the focal response to tuberculin is less marked than in any other tuberculous lesion. As we have pointed out before, the main factor in producing healing at the site of lesion is the new connective tissue formation. This is markedly stimulated during tuberculin treatment. The peculiar structure of the gland favors this formation. A too rapid stimulation by tuberculin would cause an undue formation of fibroid tissue, leaving the glands enlarged in spite of the actual healing of the tuberculous lesions. This has apparently quite an important bearing upon the question of treating tuberculous cervical adenitis, where one of the main objects is to reduce and remove, if possible, the disfiguring swellings.

The initial therapeutic dose I employ, is small enough to guarantee the absence of any visible or appreciable reaction. I will give here a few figures to demonstrate the size of the initial dose as I, as a rule, give it, using exclusively Koch's old tuberculin:

Initial Doses	O. T.	
Under 5 years	1/25000	m.g.
5 to 10 years	1/20000	"
10 to 15 years	1/15000	"
15 to 20 years	1/10000	"
Adults	1/10000	"

These doses are now gradually increased, the physician always being on the lookout for possible reaction phenomena. Personally, the author recommends a very conservative increase in dosage, as a rule limiting himself to one of 10%. Particular attention is called to the fact that the dosage is increased in a geometrical progression. The interval between doses depends upon the individual; as a rule, two doses can be administered each week. This is especially true during the first few months of treatment. Later, when the doses become larger, the interval may be lengthened to 5, 6 or 7 days, never losing sight of the individualistic character of the treatment.

How long should the tuberculin treatment be kept up? Until the patient gets well! This statement, of course, is subject to many modifications. It depends mainly upon the individual. During the course of a tuberculin treatment we see how the patient gradually is improving. He begins to look better, feel better and gain in weight. The local manifestations begin to disappear, sinuses heal and glandular swellings are reduced. Purely glandular cases respond, as a rule, to tuberculin treatment within a year. When pulmonary complications are present the duration increases. In the author's series of 270 cervical gland cases, without pulmonary involvements, the average duration of treatment was 14 months and 12 days.

The maximum dose is a variable quantity. In glandular cases I very rarely exceed one mg. It should always be remembered that tolerance to tuberculin does not mean an established immunity to tuberculosis. This tolerance can be brought about by a more rapid increase in dosage than I have recommended. But tuberculin increases the natural physiological resources of the body to fight the disease. It is our opinion that these resources are best utilized by mild stimulations by means of small doses of tuberculin, administered during a long period of time.

The value of tuberculin in the treatment of glandular tuberculosis has been pointed out time and again by various men. WILMS,[24] who has had the opportunity of seeing a great number of cases of so-called surgical tuberculosis treated with tuberculin, remarks, that tuberculin not only is suitable in the treatment of these cases, but that its use is imperative to render the organism more resistant toward the tuberculous infection, and to protect it from recurrences. His views coincide markedly with those of KRÄMER [24] who considers tuberculin the most important remedy in treating tuberculosis in children, not only the glandular lesion, but in extirpation of tuberculosis in general.

Hilus tuberculosis has received marked attention in the hands of many men. DAUTWIZ' [25] findings are of extreme interest. He studied the results of tuberculin treatment in contrast to those of hygiene and diet alone, and found how much more rapid recovery was accomplished in the former. He presented graphic illustrations of his findings by means of X-ray plates, and showed how the progressive clinical improvement corresponded to increase in fibrous tissue and encapsulation of the glands.

KRÄMER, STARK and ROHMER [24] also report good results in hilus tuberculosis.

BANDELIER and ROEPKE [23] find tuberculin of greatest value in glandular tuberculosis. They have never seen a gland break down under tuberculin treatment. Many others are quoted by them, e. g., Peiper, Jochman, Scherer, Aronade, Ullman, Dumas, Lawson, Raw, v. Ruck, Heubner, Forster and Baginski who consider tuberculin a remedy of first order.

From HAMMAN and WOLLMAN [26] may be quoted Ager, Stoll, Philip, and Griswold.

POGUE [24] and KRAUSE [24] report good results in fistulous tracts with smooth plastic scarformation.

In the author's series of 270 cases of tuberculous cervical adenitis, at the discontinuance of treatment 234 cases were apparently cured, 31 cases improved and 5 not benefited. The two latter classes all had pulmonary complications. Of the 31 improved the glandular condition had been arrested and the pulmonary lesions markedly benefited. The first class of cases—those apparently cured—included 17 that had previously been operated on, and 20 that had one or more discharging sinuses. The latter all healed, leaving very slight scars.

Subsequent examinations at the end of 6 months, 12 months and 24 months of traced cases, showed no relapse of the glandular infection during the two years following treatment. At the end of six months 51 cases had been lost track of, at the end of 12 months 83 cases, and at the end of 24 months 159 cases.

TABULATION OF ABOVE CASES

At End of Treatment

Apparently cured...................................234
Improved
    (Glandular lesions arrested, pulmonary conditions
      improved)...... 31
Not benefited.
    (Pulmonary tuberculosis).. 5

Examination 6 Months after Discontinuance of Treatment

No relapse 214
Not located. .... .51

12 Months after Treatment

No relapse....................................180
Active pulmonary tuberculosis........................2
Not located...................................83

24 Months after Treatment

No relapse....................................101
Active pulmonary tuberculosis.....................5 (3 new cases)
Not located...................................159

DILUTING OF TUBERCULIN AND PREPARATION OF DOSES

It is universally recognized that diluted solutions of tuberculin are not stable and become inactive within a few weeks. Hence, the importance of making fresh solutions.

A 1% dilution is made with sterile physiological saline solution containing ½% phenol. This solution will keep for several weeks, if kept in a cool dark place. Each 1/10 cc. of this solution contains 0.001 gm. or 1 mg. From this a series of dilutions are prepared each by 1/10 the volume strength of the former.

Dilution	Preparation	Contents of each 1/10 cc.
T.O		0.1 gm. 100 mg.
T.I 1/100	0.1 cc. T.O & 0.9 cc. diluent	0.001 gm. 1 mg.
T.II 1/1000	0.1 cc. T.I & 0.9 cc. diluent	0.0001 gm. 0.1 mg.
T.III 1/10000	0.1 cc. T.II & 0.9 cc. diluent	0.00001 gm. 0.01 mg.
T.IV 1/100,000	0.1 cc. T.III & 0.9 cc. diluent	0.000001 gm. 0.001 mg.
T.V 1/1,000,000	0.1 cc. T.IV & 0.9 cc. diluent	0.0000001 gm. 0.0001 mg.

From these dilutions any dose may be prepared. I will give you here a few tables to indicate the method.

As I have stated before, a 10% increase is recommended.

TABLE 1	TABLE 2
1.	0.2 cc.
1.100	0.22 "
1.210	0.24 "
1.331	0.26 "
1.464	0.29 "
1.610	0.32 "
1.771	0.35 "
1.948	0.39 "
2.143	0.43 "
2.357	0.47 "
2.593	0.52 "
2.853	0.57 "
3.138	0.63 "
3.452	0.69 "
3.797	0.76 "
4.177	0.84 "
4.595	0.92 "
5.054 etc.	1. "

In the above table it is shown that the 18th dose approximately represents 5 times the initial, hence the dose increases 5 times with each 17 doses. We will use 0.2 cc. as our unit of dosage. Hence, using Table 2 as our dose indicator we can increase our dose from 0.2 cc. to 1 cc., using the same dilution.

TABLE 3.

Initial Dose	18th	35th	52nd	69th	86th	103rd	
1/25000 mg.	1/5000	1/1000	1/200	1/40	1/8	5/8	108th-1 mg.
1/20000 mg.	1/4000	1/800	1/160	1/32	5/32	25/32	106th-1 mg.
1/15000 mg.	1/3000	1/600	1/120	1/24	5/24	1 mg.	(Appr.)
1/10000 mg.	1/2000	1/400	1/80	1/16	5/16	98th	(Appr.) 1 mg.

Let us now carry the initial dose of 1/25000 mg. up to 1 mg. by means of a 10% increase.

$$\frac{2}{10}\text{cc. of } T_v + \frac{8}{10}\text{cc. diluent} = \frac{10}{10} \cdot \frac{2}{10}\text{cc.} = \frac{1}{25000}\text{mg.}$$

(According to dilutions $\frac{1}{10}$cc. of T_v contains $\frac{1}{10000}$ mg. of O. T.

$\frac{2}{10}$ hence $\frac{2}{10000}$ $\frac{1}{5}$ of which is $\frac{1}{25000}$ mg.)

Using this solution for the first 18 doses, the 10% increase is insured by following Table 2. The 18th dose is 1/5000.

Using solution T_V—0.2 cc. of which contains 1/5000 mg. we proceed according to scale.

The 18th dose of this solution is 1/1000 mg., etc.

TABLE 4

					No. of Dose
0.2 cc. of T_V	+0.8 cc. dil. =	1 cc..·.0.2 cc. = 1/25000	1
Using Solution T_V		·.0.2 cc. = 1/5000	18
1 cc. of T_{IV}	+1 cc. dil. =	2 cc..·.0.2 cc. = 1/1000	35
0.25 cc. of T_{III}	+0.75 cc. dil. =	1 cc..·.0.2 cc. = 1/200	52
0.2 cc. of T_{II}	+1.4 cc. dil. =	1.6 cc..·.0.2 cc. = 1/40	69
0.1 cc. of T_I	+1.5 cc. dil. =	1.6 cc..·.0.2 cc. = 1/8	86
0.5 cc. of T_I	+1.1 cc. dil. =	1.6 cc..·.0.2 cc. = 5/8	103

Sixth dose of this latter solution equals 1 mg.

TABLE 5

				No. of Dose
0.3 cc. of T_V	+0.9 cc. dil. = 1.2 cc..·.0.2 cc. = 1/20000	1
0.2 cc. of T_{IV}	+1.4 cc. dil. = 1.6 cc..·.0.2 cc. = 1/4000	18
0.1 cc. of T_{III}	+1.5 cc. dil. = 1.6 cc..·.0.2 cc. = 1/800	35
0.1 cc. of T_{II}	+3.1 cc. dil. = 3.2 cc..·.0.2 cc. = 1/160	52
0.2 cc. of T_{II}	+1.08 cc. dil. = 1.28 cc..·.0.2 cc. = 1/32	69
0.1 cc. of T_I	+1.18 cc. dil. = 1.28 cc..·.0.2 cc. = 5/32	86
0.25 cc. of T_I	+0.39 cc. dil. = 0.64 cc..·.0.2 cc. = 25/32	103

Fourth dose of this latter solution equals approximately 1 mg.

TABLE 6

				No. of Dose
0.4 cc. of T_V	+0.8 cc. dil. = 1.2 cc..·.0.2 cc. = 1/15000	1
0.3 cc. of T_{IV}	+1.5 cc. dil. = 1.8 cc..·.0.2 cc. = 1/3000	18
0.1 cc. of T_{III}	+1.1 cc. dil. = 1.2 cc..·.0.2 cc. = 1/600	35
0.6 cc. of T_{III}	+0.84 cc. dil. = 1.44 cc..·.0.2 cc. = 1/120	52
0.3 cc. of T_{II}	+1.14 cc. dil. = 1.44 cc..·.0.2 cc. = 1/24	69
0.5 cc. of T_I	+4.3 cc. dil. = 4.8 cc..·.0.2 cc. = 5/24	86

Eighteenth dose of this solution equals approximately 1 mg.

TABLE 7

				No. of Dose
0.5 cc. of T_V	+0.5 cc. dil. = 1. cc..·.0.2 cc. = 1/10000	1
0.4 cc. of T_{IV}	+1.2 cc. dil. = 1.6 cc..·.0.2 cc. = 1/2000	18
0.2 cc. of T_{III}	+1.4 cc. dil. = 1.6 cc..·.0.2 cc. = 1/400	35
0.1 cc. of T_{II}	+1.5 cc. dil. = 1.6 cc..·.0.2 cc. = 1/80	52
0.4 cc. of T_{II}	+0.88 cc. dil. = 1.28 cc..·.0.2 cc. = 1/16	69
0.5 cc. of T_I	+2.7 cc. dil. = 3.2 cc..·.0.2 cc. = 5/16	86

Thirteenth dose of this solution approximately equals 1 mg.

X-Ray Therapy.—In more recent times the X-ray has proven to be of value in the treatment of tuberculosis of the lymph-glands, and the fact is becoming more generally recognized. During the last few years a profound study of the action of the rays, especially the deep rays, has opened new possibilities.

This has been made possible by the development of methods for measuring the rays according to which exact dosage may be administered; and also to the use of the filter, which makes it possible to use the penetrating rays necessary to affect the deeper tissues, and without which their use is impossible, because of the effect exerted upon the skin. At present it is a valuable addition to the therapeutic measures, available in treating tuberculous glands, and the use of the X-ray has been reported as satisfactory by many authors.

Produces Definite Biologic Changes.—Exposure to the Roentgen rays produces definite biologic effects. Their action is local, and because of their penetrating power the rays reach all the cells in the area treated. Inflammatory reactions often accompany the X-ray effects, especially after longer doses have been administered; but the therapeutic effect is dependent upon the specific effect, although the healing process may be aided by the inflammation.

Effect of Exposure.—The tissue cells vary in regard to their sensitiveness to the X-ray, those most affected being the ones that are rich in protoplasm and with active metabolism. The more highly specialized cells are affected first; pathological tissues composed of young and rapidly growing cells of low vitality offer little resistance to the rays. The more embryonal in type is the cell, the more easily it is destroyed, as is evidenced by the effect exerted upon such tissues as sarcomata, which cells are typically embryonal and very sensitive. Cells of diseased tissue are more sensitive than are healthy ones, and hyperemic tissues are more affected than anemic ones. Round celled infiltrations are easily destroyed, while connective tissue is affected with difficulty. Lymphoid cells are very susceptible to the Roentgen rays.

Has a Selective Action.—The favorable influence of Roentgen therapy in tuberculosis of the lymphatic glands is due in large part to this selective action of the rays upon the lymphoid tissue of the glands, since this tissue is in a state of chronic inflammation and attended by proliferative changes. These cells are destroyed and replaced by fibrous tissue cells, as can be demonstrated at operation, or by microscopical examination. The lymphatic channels also become converted into fibrous tissue, thus eliminating the possibility of further spread of the disease and isolating it in the lymph-nodes, where it is finally overcome. This destructive effect upon the lymphatic element, as upon all cells which have a marked faculty of proliferation, is the most pronounced action observed. The growth of connective tissue cells is stimulated and cicatrization follows.

Action Distinctive to Giant Cells.—According to Pirie [27] an important factor is the destruction, by the rays, of the rapidly developing giant cells. Sections of the giant cells, observed in microscopic preparations, often show tubercle bacilli, and he believes that these cells become inactive and constitute a place where the bacilli can live unharmed by the leucocytes. By the destruction of these cells the bacilli are deprived of this protection, and can then be destroyed by the leucocytes. With this in view he makes use of the maximum dose the skin will stand, at intervals of a week. This dose destroys the giant cells, which may form in a week's time, and this same dose according to Pirie, only stimulates the attacking leucocytes. The question arises, whether the Roentgen rays have any direct action on the tubercle bacillus. This is usually considered as a negligible factor; and experiments upon guinea-pigs, quoted by Broca and Mahar,[28] seem to invalidate any such hypothesis.

Effect on the Opsonic Index.—There are some grounds for believing that irradiation may produce serological changes in the organism so treated. This may account for the observation occasionally made of the disease in size of neighboring or distant similarly affected glands, when treatment is directed to tuberculous cervical glands. The systematic effect has also been studied by its effect upon the opsonic index. It has been shown that the index rises as treatment progresses, but that it will fall into the negative phase and the progress of healing will be retarded, if treatment is too severe. The opsonic index changes more slowly and does not show such sudden variations as are caused by tuberculin. These facts show, that the treatment must begin intelligently and proper dosage be administered, if the best results are to be obtained. If the dosage is too large a general reaction may result, evidently due to changes in the blood serum or to toxemia resulting from tissue destruction.

KIENBOECK [29] attributes the destruction of cells to a recession of metabolic activity. RICHARD has studied the effect of the X-ray upon enzyme action and found that slight exposures increased enzyme action, while greater exposures were inhibitive or destructive. He believes that the direct injury to the chromation of the cells is undoubtedly important, but that changes in enzyme action, resulting from the action of the rays, likewise plays a considerable part in the resulting injury.

Healing Action.—The action of the Roentgen rays in producing healing in tuberculous glands is then dependent upon several factors. They bring about actual destruction of the tuberculous granulation tissue, as has been uniformly demonstrated by the microscopic examination of irradiated tubercles. Epithelioid and giant cells become degenerated, shrunken and finally disintegrated and are replaced by a proliferation of fibroblasts, which are stimulated by the rays. The rays also cause a certain amount of reaction in the surrounding tissues, resulting in hyperemia and crowding of the vessels surrounding the lesion with leucocytes, which promote absorption of the inflammatory products, and in infiltration of the tissues with small round cells, which wall off the diseased areas by connective tissue formation and thus favor healing. The theories have also been proposed, that the X-rays have an autotuberculin or autovaccin effect due to the liberation of tuberculin by degeneration of the tubercles, or that the effect upon the bacilli may lessen the toxin formation, or bring about a chemical change in the toxin.

A Valuable Therapeutic Agent.—The X-ray is a valuable therapeutic agent, whether used alone or, better, combined with tuberculin treatment. It is preferable to surgical treatment over which it possesses numerous advantages. It can be used to great advantage in those cases where the poor nutrition of a patient may preclude operative interference. It is painless and avoids the shock and the dangers of an extensive dissection of the glands which often requires a long and tedious operation. The glands are reduced to hard fibrous nodules and the lymphatic channels, by means of which the tuberculous infection spreads from gland to gland, are transformed into fibrous cords.

Protective Action.—This sclerosis of blood and lymphatic vessels, in the area subjected to irradiation, is the best safeguard against the further spread of infection. Furthermore, the penetrating power of the rays enable them to thoroughly reach all diseased glands in the irradiated area, thereby treating glands that may be overlooked by the operator in making an excision. Roentgen therapy also treats effecitvely those glands which are infected but show no enlargement or other visible evidence of their infection. By some the X-ray is used in conjunction with surgery and may be considered as a valuable aid. If a radical operation is done, the use of the-X-ray following operation may lessen the chances of recurrences, and in incomplete operations the rays may then effect a complete cure. In advanced cases with sinuses and with matting of the tissues a radical operation may be precluded, and in such cases the X-ray may heal the sinuses and promote a cure. If the cases are seen early the scars of healed sinuses or operations may be avoided and a perfect cosmetic effect obtained, the tanning of the skin disappearing in due time. With Roentgen therapy the patient does not need to be confined to a hospital, and can be following out the proper hygiènic and dietetic régime.

The Technique.—The technique employed by various Roentgenologists differs in its details, but the principles involved are the same. I shall not discuss the technique of Roentgen therapy in detail, for it may be found in works devoted to that subject. The effect is produced by the rays absorbed, and the object of treatment should, therefore, be to cause the greatest possible absorption of rays by the diseased tissues. This does not imply that we should employ the highest possible doses, but that the highest possible concentration of rays should be upon the diseased tissue, with the minimum of absorption where it is not desired. Since the skin is the most exposed tissue, the problem is to produce an effect upon the underlying tissues without injury to the integument. To obtain this result a tube with a penetration of Number 6 Benoist, producing hard rays, is employed. They have a maximum penetrating power and are absorbed to the least degree by the skin. But the most satisfactory results cannot be obtained by this method alone; and in addition to this, a filter must be employed to absorb the soft rays, which have little penetrating power and are absorbed by the skin. For this purpose various substances are interposed between the tube and the skin to intercept the passage of the soft rays; some workers use a plate of aluminum 1 to 2 mm. thick; others employ tin foil, or sole leather. The exposed area should extend wide of the disease and the surrounding tissues be protected by lead foil. In the neck the entire region, from the mastoid process above down to and including the apex of the lung, should be subjected to irradiation.

Dose Employed.—The dosage employed also varies, some preferring a massive dose at long intervals, and others, smaller doses more frequently repeated. The best results are obtained when the dosage is accurate: it should, therefore, be controlled by Sabourand's pastilles, or other methods of measuring the quantity of rays applied to the affected area.

Erythema Dose.—KIENBOECK [30] employed a hard tube, with a penetration above Benoist Number 6, at a distance of 20 to 30 cm., and a filter of aluminum, glass or hard leather. When possible, he irradiates from various sides or angles. This so-called "cross-firing" method is advantageous, for the diseased area may be treated and a different skin area exposed each time, thus obtaining the maximum absorption of rays where it is desired, and with minimum damage to the integument. He usually applies the maximum superficial dose, called also the erythema, normal or epilation dose; and repeats it in three or four weeks, continuing treatment over months until cure is accomplished. Giving maximal doses at one sitting permits of more accurate control of the dose. Where the application of the rays necessitates the use of a greater skin distance and harder rays, he commends a modified method and divides the maximal dose over succeeding days, or gives one-third the full dose every eight to fourteen days.

PIRIE [29] employs a filter and gives one-third the dose required to produce epillation, as measured by Sabourand's pastilles, at intervals of a week.

HUBENY's method consists of the administration of one-half an erythema dose, seven to eight Wehnult, plus four mm. of aluminum, repeated three successive times at two weeks intervals, then twice at three weeks intervals, gradually increasing the intervals between treatments until about eight treatments have been given.

H. MOWAT [31] employs rays obtained by the use of a hard tube and current of two or three milliampèremeters and a filter of 1.5 mm. of aluminum. He gives an exposure of at least one full Sabourand dose once or twice weekly.

Dose for Children.—O. H. PETERSEN [32] irradiates with hard rays obtained by means of an aluminum filter 3 mm. thick, thereby securing much better and more uniform depth, action, and better skin protection. As a single dose for adults and older children be employs one-half of the maximal dose. For younger children he diminishes the dose according to age. He repeats the dose in the beginning every four weeks, and in the further course of the treatment, allows longer intervals between exposures.

TIXIER [33] applies 3½ Holzknecht units every eight to fourteen days.

TONSEY [34] states that tuberculous glands are readily amenable to treatment by a radiance with penetration of Benoist Number 5 or Number 6. He gives short applications of about 1–½ minutes at a distance of 9 inches from the anticathode, three times a week until some reaction appears, when the treatment should be intermitted. Each application should be calculated to be a little less than one Holzknecht unit. Another plan is to make massive application of 4 or 5 H. units at a single session, or two or more within the course of two or three weeks.

Dangers.—There are certain dangers attending the use of the X-ray, and it should be employed only by one skilled in its application for therapeutic purposes. The treatment is often stretched out over a long period of time, and the cumulative effect of the rays must be avoided, for it may produce severe reaction and injury to the skin at a remote time, although each individual dose has been below the border of danger. According to ISELIN [35] the danger border for the neck lies at about six full Sabourand doses filtered through one mm. of aluminum. A common experience is the diminution of the glandular swellings as a result of the late action of the rays. Hence, in difficult cases six exposures of maximal dosage may be given at intervals of one month followed by an interval of several months to await the late action of the rays.

The Local Reaction.—Following exposure there is a local reaction in the glands. It occurs very soon and lasts for a variable period of time. It may be very slight or consist in swelling of the glands and painfulness in the treated area. The discomfort is usually not so very marked. With the more massive doses there may be, in addition, a general reaction characterized by malaise, nausea and vomiting appearing soon after the exposure. Such reactions call for a more careful regulation of the dose.

Valuable in Earlier Stages.—As with other methods of treatment, Roentgen therapy is especially indicated in the early stages of the disease before caseation and suppuration have occurred. The most favorable cases for treatment are those which are not so far advanced, especially in children and young adults, where the glands are palpable as firm hyperplastic nodules. In the later stage, where the glands have become adherent forming a mass, the first effect of treatment noted is a lessening of the periadenitis, and the glands that were agglomerated become isolated. Hyperplastic glands enlarge after an exposure to the Roentgen ray; later they decrease markedly in size, the extent to which they subside depending upon their previous state of inflammation. The retrogression may be sufficient to cause complete disappearance of the nodes, but more often the glands persist as small palpable innocuous fibroid nodules, which never entirely disappear. X-ray therapy is not confined to the earlier forms, although it is in these that the best results are obtained. Older glands which are about to undergo caseation, or in which caseation has begun, are less favorable to treat and softening is often hastened. Aspiration or incision are then required to remove the pus, after which treatment may be resumed. Tonsey has observed excellent results from the use of the X-ray in suppurating tuberculous glands, opened spontaneously or by the surgeon's knife.

Fistulæ do not Yield.—The ulcerating and fistulous forms are the most difficult and the least favorable for treatment. Secondary infection is usually present, but in spite of this the fistulæ may close up, the ulcers heal, the glandular swellings disappear, the infiltration becomes less in amount, and the discharge changes from a purulent to a serious character. The fistulæ close with difficulty after prolonged treatment, but leave better scars than those cases healing spontaneously.

Patients with repeated occurrences after operation, or in whom ulcerations and sinuses still persist, can be successfully treated. With a subsidence of the local disease the general health of the patient improves, his appetite returns, and he gains in weight and strength.

In the hands of Roentgenologists, who have used an accurately measured dosage, we find uniform reports of success with a large percentage of cures and a scarcity of recurrences.

Views of Investigators.—Philipowicz[36] finds the X-ray most satisfactory in treating tuberculous adenitis. He finds that at least six months' time is necessary for treatment. The nodes subsided completely or remained as small dense fibroid nodules. Fistulæ healed with flexible scars.

Iselin[37] reports 206 cases of glandular tuberculosis treated with the X-ray with complete cure in 133, and improvement in all but 4 cases.

Roques[38] considers the X-ray to be the treatment of choice.

O. H. Petersen[39] concludes, that no glandular tuberculosis is absolutely refractile to treatment with the X-ray, but advises that it be combined with other measures and not used alone.

BROCA and MAHAR [28] report 79 cases, 45 of which were open and suppurating. In 36 cases they obtained complete healing. In 24, marked improvement, and in 19 there was some improvement but treatment was interrupted. They never used over six exposures and found that incision of the softened glands was of value in hurrying the healing.

FRITSCH [40] submitted 33 cases to this treatment. In the absence of tuberculosis elsewhere he considers the treatment very effectual. He sees advantages in combining 6 months of X-ray with other treatment.

Good results have been reported by BLAISCH,[41] MOWAT,[31] TONSEY,[34] VON MUTSENBACHER,[42] BERGONIE [43] and others.

TONSEY [34] considers tuberculous mediastinal glands amenable to treatment by Roentgenotherapy. He employs a radiance with an intensity of Benoist Number 6; the anticathode is placed 13 inches from the chest and a piece of sole leather, or an aluminum filter, to intercept the soft rays. He gives exposures of 3 minutes' duration twice a week with intermissions on the development of some erythema of the skin. Massive doses, he believes, are less desirable than milder, frequently repeated ones. The results are variable, but it is capable of great benefit in certain cases.

Surgical Treatment.—Tuberculosis of the lymphatic glands has always been classed under the heading of "Surgical Tuberculosis," and various surgical procedures have been advised and employed in its treatment. The surgical treatment must vary according to the pathological conditions which present themselves as indications for treatment. All gland groups are not amenable to surgical intervention; for example, the bronchial glands, by reason of their deep-seated location within the thorax, cannot be reached by the knife. Various procedures are classed under the heading of surgical treatment, and we shall consider excision, aspiration, incision, currettement, and injections into the glands.

Excision.—Under the heading of excision of tuberculous lymph-glands, I shall first consider the so-called radical operation which aims at the cure of tuberculosis by eliminating from the organism all infected glands by means of an extensive dissection. As an example of this method of procedure, we may discuss the well-known operation for tuberculous cervical nodes. This operation was formerly used extensively and no class of cases was considered more within the realm of the surgeon's care.

At the present time the ideas of surgical treatment of this condition are becoming more and more conservative, and attention is being turned to methods of treatment, such as we have outlined above, rather than to extensive dissections. This I consider as an advancement in our methods of treatment of glandular tuberculosis, and although there are surgeons who still advise and employ methods of dissection, I believe them to be contraindicated and productive of poorer results than conservative and specific treatment. I shall not consider the technique in detail; this may be found in works on surgery. An incision is made either parallel to the natural folds of skin in the neck, or along the margin of the Sterno-cleido-mastoid muscle. The incisions must be free, for the glandular involvement is extensive, always more so than it appears to be from external examination. Flaps of skin and the Platysma muscle are reflected and the field exposed. Then by the knife and blunt dissection the surgeon attempts to remove, as completely as possible, all infected glands without injury to the many important structures found in the neck. The operation is difficult, to say the least, and can only be performed thoroughly by a well-qualified surgeon. The operation is often a lengthy one as time and care are required in freeing infected glands which are adherent to the internal jugular vein, or imbedded firmly about important nerves. Glands are often ruptured in removal and infectious material contaminates the wound. The operation means the loss of more or less blood. If the operation is performed with an aseptic technique, healing readily occurs with the usual scar at the site of incision.

Operation Serious in Children.—The operation is not a trivial one to be undertaken lightly, and it is attended by a certain risk. Many of the cases presenting themselves for treatment are in children who, as the result of their long-standing tuberculous infection, are anæmic and poorly nourished. Such children are very sensitive to the loss of blood and unless proper attention has been paid to preliminary treatment, death may ensue. Surgeons, however, are familiar with the value of this preoperative treatment in building up the strength of the patient, increasing the resistance, improving his nutrition and raising his hemoglobin index, and the mortality in the hands of experienced men has not been high. Surgeons also recognize the necessity of subsequent or post-operative treatment in these cases. In my opinion if these general measures were but combined with tuberculin therapy, properly administered, the surgical part of the treatment might be largely dispensed with.

Infected Glands may not all be Enlarged.—We must consider the possibility of the removal by dissection of all the diseased glands, for the conception of the operation is based upon the opinion, that by timely operative interference the foci of infection may be removed. We should remember that the glandular infection is always more extensive than it appears to be, and the lymphatic glands of the region of the neck are especially numerous. Very often we see a fine multiple enlargement of the cervical nodes. BARTELS and others have shown that glands may be infected and show no pathological changes, the infection being demonstrable only by animal inoculation. It is to be seen that such glands might easily be overlooked in making an extensive dissection in a case presenting a multiple spreading involvement of the nodes. A radical removal by dissection of all diseased glands may, therefore, be considered an impossibility.

Bronchial Glands also may be Enlarged.—The possibility of the presence of tuberculosis elsewhere must be borne in mind. Careful examination often reveals infected bronchial glands, or a pulmonary involvement. In such cases the infection of the cervical lymphatic glands is but a part of the tuberculous infection, from which the individual is suffering, and operative treatment of these glands may reduce the patient's resistance to such an extent that the other foci may increase their activity, and the result be disastrous. We are too prone to consider tuberculous glands simply as a chronic adenopathy rather than as a manifestation of tuberculosis. Surely it is just as important to recognize and treat tuberculosis as such, when it affects the lymphatic glands, as when it affects other organs of the body. I consider tuberculosis of the lymphatic glands as a medical disease and treat it as such.

In surgical treatment, by means of a radical operation, the only glands treated are those which have been removed. The immediate results, as far as the disfigurement caused by a large mass of glands is concerned, is usually satisfactory and in some cases the operation may fairly be described as successful. But in numerous instances, the effect of the operation can only be a partial one, from the nature of the pathological condition with which we are dealing, for it is obviously impossible to remove all the infected glands. Even when the manifestly diseased glands have been removed, the final cure is brought about in the same way as with general hygienic and specific treatment. The amount of infection with which the patient is contending is diminished, but the surgical procedure has not eradicated his tuberculosis. There can scarcely be a doubt that the cure of tuberculosis by any one method of treatment is, in the end, brought about by the natural processes of healing. We must, therefore, employ those measures which will be of greatest aid to these natural healing processes.

Operations May Assist.—We must, therefore, consider the question of radical operation, not as a means of absolute cure, but merely as an adjunct to our methods of treatment and question if this removal of the part of the infected tissue, by means of a mutilating operation, is the best means at our command for assisting the organism to combat its tuberculosis. The combination of general hygiene and tuberculin treatment, as I have outlined, aims at the increase of the resistance of the body to tuberculous infection by the development of toximmunity, and a stimulation of the factors of healing. In tuberculin treatment we are treating every gland that may be infected with tuberculosis, as well as tuberculous foci elsewhere in the body, if such happen to exist as they not infrequently do. In the surgical treatment the glands which have been removed are the only ones treated. The very success of the operative treatment in some cases has diverted attention from the tuberculous infection as such, and the final result in many cases has, therefore, been disappointing. The mutilating operation cannot but lower the local and general resistance to infection, in this respect being opposed to tuberculin therapy. In numerous instances, in which the operation has seemed immediately successful, disfiguring enlargement has recurred and not infrequently with suppuration, and often have I observed cases where, after repeated operations, enlargement of the glands continued to reappear with a gradual extension of the infection downward and more deeply. I have seen many cases in which an extensive operation has been performed for deep lying diseased glands, and where little relief has followed, or the disfigurement of the group of glands removed was soon replaced by enlargement of another group, often those on the opposite side of the neck. (See Plates XI and XII). I have had cases present themselves to me for treatment with a large mass of glands, causing great disfigurement and ill health, who gave a history and showed the scars of three or four operations. After having submitted to repeated operations these patients still had their tuberculous glands, because all those infected had not been removed and there had not been sufficient treatment directed to the assistance of the natural processes of healing. In such cases the infection has subsided, and the glandular enlargement gradually disappeared, not to recur under the influence of tuberculin properly administered. The physician is frequently called upon to treat these cases which have not been cured by radical operation. I, therefore, believe it is safer and wiser to make use of the same treatment in tuberculous glands that we would institute in other forms of tuberculosis. The value of tuberculin cannot be denied, and many clinicians will testify to its use in the treatment of tuberculous adenitis.

Value of Early Operation.—Surgeons favor early operation before caseation and suppuration have occurred. Surely the best results are to be obtained by any method of treatment when it is applied early. After caseation and suppuration have occurred, surgical measures may become necessary, as tuberculin will not do the impossible, namely, remove the necrotic tissue.

But simpler measures than a radical operation suffice in these cases of suppuration and abscess formation. One of the arguments for early surgical intervention is to prevent the occurrence of suppuration, but it must be admitted that this is not the usual termination of all cases of tuberculosis of the lymphatic glands. In cases allowed to run their course probably only about one-half terminate in suppuration. When properly treated and treatment instituted early, suppuration may be considered as an incidental occurrence and it is relatively uncommon when we consider the large number of glands usually infected and showing infiltration. Yet in advocating radical surgical treatment, attention has been chiefly centered upon this incidental occurrence and too little upon the tuberculous infection per se. Rational treatment should, therefore, be directed to the essential factor, the tuberculous infection, rather than to the condition of suppuration, which does not necessarily occur. Failure of surgical treatment has resulted by direction of attention from the more important factor, and the result has been a limitation of operative treatment and more attention to specific treatment and hygienic measures destined to bring about healing in a natural way. I believe, therefore, that we should institute such treatment which, of itself, is prophylactic against suppuration. While surgical removal of suppurating glands may be satisfactory, it is uncertain and gives no assurance that the other glands, likewise infected, which have not been removed, will not soon be in the same condition as the ones removed. Tuberculous glands are amenable to tuberculin treatment, and if suppuration should occur, or be found when the case first presents itself for treatment, the pus may be removed by the simple method described below, the condition being still medical, not surgical.

Tuberculin Treatment Leaves no Scars.—The radical operation has been favored by some on the grounds that the scar left by operation is much less disfiguring than those resulting from the healing of fistulæ resulting from the rupture and discharge of suppurating glands. But this argument presupposes that suppuration is inevitable, and can be remedied in no other way which, as we have shown, is far from being the case if the patients present themselves before abscesses have ruptured. If suppuration does occur it can be treated by aspiration, as outlined below, and no fistulæ need result, and an extensive dissection is unnecessary. It is surely better, as far as cosmetic results are obtained, to treat a case so that no scar at all results than to have a scar, the result of an operation, even though it be only slightly disfiguring. (See Plate XIII.) And when we consider that some cases may have several scars from repeated operations, and still have a large mass of suppurating glands, I do not think operation is justifiable on the grounds that it will cure and leave a less unsightly scar.

The length of time required for tuberculin treatment is necessarily longer than when surgical treatment is employed. But tuberculin treatment is not merely directed against a few glands in one area, which are manifestly tuberculous, but against all infected glands, or other tuberculous foci, in the body, and when favorable result has been obtained, the possibility of a further extension of the disease has been largely removed. But since surgical measures do not, in any way, prevent recurrence but expose the patient to the advent of tuberculosis elsewhere, and since the knife must always leave a certain amount of mutilation, I believe these measures should be entirely replaced by judiciously administered tuberculin therapy, combined with general hygienic and dietetic measures and other useful adjuncts to treatment, such as heliotherapy and the X-ray, when they are available. In addition, we should clean up the portals of entry to prevent added infection.

Results.—In a recent article Dowd gives the following results in 687 cases treated by operation by himself, or his associates and assistants. He divides his cases into groups:

Group 1.—In this group he classes the early stages of infection with involvement of the upper cervical lymphatic glands. There were 452 patients in this group. Their average age was 8.03 years. They were observed for variable periods of time; 67 were followed from six to twenty years; 23 were followed into the sixth year; 36 into the fifth year; 53 into the fourth year; 61 into the

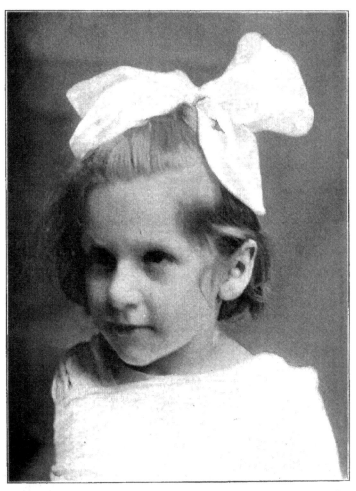

PLATE XIII.—Tuberculosis of the cervical glands in a child. Age 6. Showing typical results following tuberculin treatment.

third year; 65 into the second year and 49 into the first year; 98 were not observed after leaving the hospital; 91% of the cases traced were apparently cured when last seen; 9.75% showed slight evidence of recurrence; 1 patient had died of typhoid fever; 8% had secondary operations during the periods of observation.

Group 2.—In this group are included cases with abscesses and sinuses and involvement of glands along the entire jugular chain and the anterior border of the Trapezius muscle. One hundred and eighty-five patients were included in this group, the average age was 15.9 years, and 69 were over 20 years. Twenty-nine of these patients were followed from six to twenty years; 11 were followed into the sixth year; 18 into the fifth year; 14 into the fourth year; 24 into the third year; 19 into the second year and 10 into the first year; 60 were not observed after leaving the hospital. 68.2 per cent of the patients traced were apparently cured when last seen; 23.8% showed recurrences when last seen; 5.5% had died of intercurrent disease, partly tuberculous; 2.4% or 3 patients died in the hospital; 28.5% of the traced patients had two or more operations.

Group 3.—This group included those with diffuse tuberculosis, the patients showing little resistance to tuberculosis, the neck infection quickly involving a great number of nodes, and there were usually evidences of tuberculosis elsewhere. There were 50 patients in this group, and their average age was 12.7 years; 13 of these patients were followed from six to seventeen years; 3 were followed into the sixth year; 5 into the fifth year; 2 into the fourth year; 5 into the third year; 9 into the second year, and 6 into the first year; 34% of the patients traced were suffering from recurrence or other forms of tuberculosis; 20.4% had died of intercurrent disease, largely tuberculosis; 1 died in the hospital after a minor palliative operation.

These statistics may be taken as a fair average of the results obtained by radical operation.

Currettement of the glands by means of an incision and scraping out of the caseous masses is inferior to, and even less to be advised, than is excision of the diseased glands, but is employed by some in advanced cases where excision is impossible.

Suppurating Glands Should be Aspirated.—The treatment of suppurating glands should be instituted early before they rupture and the adjacent tissues become involved. The indication is to remove the pus in the simplest possible manner, and softened glands may be treated by aspiration or incision. I, personally, employ aspiration. The technique is simple. The skin is cleansed with soap and water and alcohol, or tincture of iodine applied. A local anesthetic may be used for anesthetizing the skin, if it is desired. A needle should be selected with a calibre of sufficient size to permit the withdrawal of pus, which is often thick and curdy. Aspiration is effected by means of a syringe. The needle is inserted into the softened gland at an angle and through the healthy skin and subcutaneous tissues, rather than directly over the gland at a point where rupture is threatening. By so doing the healthy tissues will contract and the needle track will quickly heal and no sinus will result, as might be the case if the needle were inserted at the point of threatened rupture where the skin is thinned, its nutrition impaired, and contraction of the needle track prevented by the adhesions to the underlying tissues. One aspiration may suffice, or it may be necessary to repeat it several times, inserting the needle at different points each time. Under tuberculin the glandular enlargement then usually subsides and rupture and sinus formation is prevented.

Injections into the Glands.—Injections into the glands have been employed by many from time to time, and a vast number of substances have been employed for the purpose. Injections into infiltrated glands are not to be advised. After removal of the pus from a softened gland by aspiration, injections into the abscess cavity are employed by some, and iodoform in oil or glycerin has been perhaps the most extensively used.

An incision for the purpose of evacuating the pus, contained in a softened gland, may be employed, but is less preferable than aspiration. Observing the usual aseptic precautions, a small incision is made into the gland and the pus evacuated. The lining of the abscess cavity may be scraped with a curette,

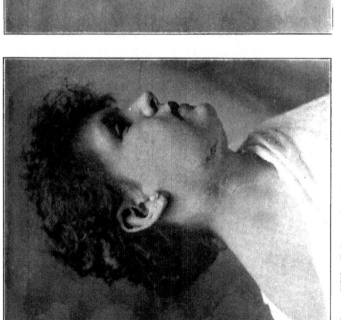

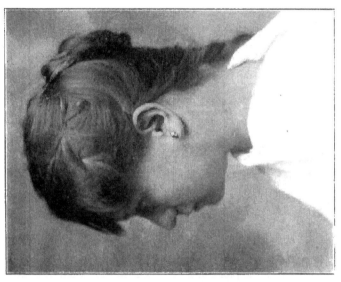

PLATE XIV.—Tuberculosis of the submaxillary and cervical glands. Scars following surgical treatment.

PLATE XV.—Typical markings following surgical treatment of tuberculosis lymphadenitis.

and the wound closed by sutures. Iodoform emulsion may, or may not, be injected into abscess cavities so treated.

Heliotherapy.—The use of sunlight as a therapeutic agent in the treatment of various maladies dates back to an early period of time. In more recent years solar energy, as well as artificial light, has come into prominence as a remedial agent, largely through the work of FINSEN. In addition to sunlight, the Roentgen ray and the quartz light have an important place in treatment.

Heliotherapy in the treatment of tuberculosis has been most extensively employed by and yielded the best results in the hands of ROLLIER. In 1903 he established at Leysin, Switzerland, a sanitorium for the exclusive sunlight treatment of surgical forms of tuberculosis. Leysin is situated in the Alps at a height of 4,000 feet above the sea level. The climatic conditions, characterized by intense sunlight, dry atmosphere, free from dust and insects, but little wind, a moderate warmth in summer and not too great cold in winter, admit of insolation in both seasons with uninterrupted open air life. The buildings are protected from winds, and the beds are placed on the balconies in the sunshine.

Method of Application.—The treatment is begun with gradual exposures, at first for only a short interval, and repeated several times a day. The feet are first exposed, then the legs, thighs, pelvis, abdomen and thorax, the latter being reached at the end of about seven or eight days. The length of time of the exposures and their frequency are gradually increased until the entire body is pigmented, and then general exposures of the naked body are given. The eyes are protected from the direct rays of the sun and by the gradual exposure to the sun's rays, pigmentation occurs without the production of a dermatitis solarum, or other discomfort to the patient. The intensity of the sunlight in the higher altitudes is much greater than at lower levels, especially during the winter months. There is a marked difference in the sun and shade temperatures. When there is snow on the ground the thermometer may register 0° C. in the shade and 50° to 60° in the sunshine.

The Ultraviolet Rays.—The volume of the ultraviolet rays of the sunlight increases with the higher level of altitude. The difference in the intensity of these rays in summer and winter is comparatively small at the high altitude, but is great at a low level.

Theory of the Action.—It is not yet possible to explain the exact nature of the mechanism of the reaction of the tissues to the exposure to sunlight. Both the invisible and the visible rays doubtless perform definite therapeutic functions. The visible rays furnish a factor of warmth, and from the invisible are derived the chemical effects of the actinic or ultraviolet rays.

Effects of Exposure.—Some of the effects of the exposure to sunlight, which are noted clinically, may be considered. The first effect noted is a hypertrophy of the skin. There is an increase in the pigmentation and in the growth of hair. Pigmentation is believed to play an important rôle in the treatment. It is believed that it lowers the resistance of the skin to the passage of the light rays and modifies the heat rays so as to remove their harmful effects. The hypertrophy increases the vitality and resistance of the skin, affording added protection from the cold. ROLLIER regards early advent of pigmentation as prognostic of good results. He has observed that the rapidity of healing of the disease is proportionate to the degree of pigmentation and that blondes were less responsive and required longer treatment.

More recently JESIONEK [44] has stated, that he considers the pigment to be the main factor in the therapeutic action of light as applied in heliotherapy. He considers that the effect observed in this method of treatment is due, not to the pigment retained in the cells, but to the excess which is formed and thrown off by the cells. He assumes that certain substances are formed as products of the special activity of the skin, in consequence of the action of light, and believes that the excess of these substances gets into the circulation and reaches the tuberculous focus.

Rapid Absorption of Pigment.—That pigment can be rapidly absorbed, is proven by the whitening of tanned skins when no longer exposed to sunlight. Negroes removed from their natural environment no longer generate pigment in abundance, and JESIONEK believes that the system may feel the lack of this pigment to which the cells have become accustomed and asks if this might not be one of the possible causes for the susceptibility to tuberculosis of the negro race in civilization. He states that among whites individuals of a pronounced brunette type, and hence with a greater pigment-producing power, acquire tuberculosis less frequently than blondes. For these and other reasons he ascribes to the melanotic pigment of the skin great importance in the success of heliotherapy.

Effect on Metabolism.—The Metabolism is raised. The dry mountain air is invigorating, the appetite is stimulated, and the activity of the organs of the body is increased. Increased metabolism increases the bodily resistance to infection and stimulates the natural healing process, which are essential for the cure of any tuberculous lesion.

The Hemoglobin Index is raised, and the number of erythrocytes is increased. It is a familiar observation that the latter occurs with residence at a high altitude. The sunlight has a vasomotor excitant effect upon the circulation of the skin, which reacts on the internal circulation.

The cool dry mountain air has a stimulant effect on the nervous system, and the respirations are increased in depth. The exposure to sunlight produces a local hyperemia which has a desirable effect on the lesions, increasing their blood supply and flooding them with antibodies and leucocytes, thus favoring their healing.

Ultraviolet rays have a bactericidal effect, but in heliotherapy it is probably a negligible factor. On dark days treatment with the X-ray or the Cooper Hewitt light is substituted by ROLLIER.

Effect of the Treatment.—The effect of the treatment cannot be considered as a local one, except to a very slight degree. We must suppose that the general condition of the body is strengthened through stimulation of the metabolism and that, as a consequence, the body is put in a position to overcome the disease and bring about healing. The benefit of the high altitude, the stimulant effect of the cool dry air and the effects on the blood, all probably have something to do with the success of the treatment.[45]

Rollier's Success.—ROLLIER has treated all kinds of tuberculous gland cases, from the simple uncomplicated ones to the suppurating type of the fistulæ, a complete recovery is the rule. In cases of suppurating glands the pus formation is at first increased but later is followed by drying up of the discharge and healing of the fistulæ. In addition to the exposure to the sun and dietetic measures, the children receive cod liver oil. An attempt is made to prevent the formation of sinuses, abscesses are aspirated and injected with iodoform in oil or glycerin. When not exposed to the sun, sinuses are covered with an alcohol dressing to prevent secondary infection. Six months to two years are required for treatment of gland cases. In cases where sinuses form, the scars are, as a rule, less disfiguring than in cases treated by a radical operation.[46] HIRSCH [47] quotes the following statistics of tuberculous lymph-nodes:

```
88 cases —
        81 cured
         6 improved
         1 died
```

The Disadvantages.—There are many disadvantages to ROLLIER's sunlight treatment, which prevent its general adoption in the treatment of tuberculosis of the lymphatic glands. A high altitude is required and in this respect, and in the other essential climatic conditions of intense sunlight, dry air and little wind, only certain localities are available. The number of patients must necessarily be limited for this and other reasons. At lower levels there are fewer sunny days, and the volume of the ultraviolet rays is less and is more variable. The greater humidity of the air absorbs a portion of the actinic rays.

WEBB [48] has carried out ROLLIER's method of treatment for three years at Colorado Springs. He finds it to be of much benefit in the treatment of surgical tuberculosis—bones, joints and glands, but is not as optimistic about it as ROLLIER. He warns against the careless employment of sun baths without medical control, as harm can be done by them.

That exclusive sunlight treatment cannot be adopted at low

levels and in ordinary climates, where the weather conditions are uncertain and vary from one extreme to another, is evident. The value of sunlight, however, cannot be contested. Animal experiments have shown that animals exposed to light were more resistant to infection than those kept in the dark. The detrimental effect of the depressing influence of living in dark habitations, as do many of the poor in our large cities, is a well-known fact. We may, therefore, urge an outdoor life to those who are infected with tuberculosis, and in fact we should urge all individuals to spend as much time as possible in the fresh air and sunshine if they would be healthy.

In the treatment of tuberculosis of the lymphatic glands, we may employ more intensive applications of actinic rays than are obtained in sunlight alone, by the use of the Roentgen rays or the ultraviolet rays obtained from an arc, quartz or mercury vapor light.

Ocean and Mountain Climates.—The temperature of ocean climates varies less according to latitude than inland climates. Sea air is pure and free from dust and pathogenic microorganisms. It is moist and equable, its evenness being characteristic. These characters give to the ocean climate a sedative and relaxing effect upon the nervous system. As sea air is at its maximum density the volume of each inspiration contains relatively a larger quantity of oxygen and leads to increased depth and slowing of the respirations. The mucous membranes and skin are more active, and the sea air is a stimulant to nutrition and metabolism. The appetite is increased, the digestion stimulated, muscular strength is augmented and the red blood-cells and hemoglobin and body weight are increased. It has long been recognized that tuberculous gland cases do well at the seaside resorts, and an ocean climate is expressly indicated in glandular tuberculosis when the lungs are not also affected. In addition sea baths are available at ocean resorts. Sea bathing was advised and its value recognized in glandular tuberculosis by the older physicians. A number of factors contribute to the therapeutic value of sea baths. Besides the stimulating effect to the skin exerted by the salt water, the cooler temperature acts as a thermic stimulus and increases metabolism as is visible in a keener appetite and increased weight.

As a means for stimulating metabolism the indications for sea bathing are the same as those for sea climate and air. They are excellent for the fairly robust individuals, who are able to withstand strong impulses, but are unsuitable for anæmic weak patients who cannot react properly. The frequency and the duration of sea baths will depend upon the reactive capacity of the individual. When sea bathing is not available some results may be obtained from salt water baths at home.

Mountain climates are likewise of value in the treatment of glandular tuberculosis. At high altitudes the air is pure and free from organisms and of less density than at lower levels. The air is cool and dry and the sunshine is abundant. The cardiac and respiratory functions, the nervous system, and general metabolism are stimulated and the number of red blood-cells increased. For more robust patients the climate is valuable but if patients are not robust, but weak and anæmic, the stimulating effect may be harmful.

Soap Treatment.—Friction with soft or green soap was, according to CORNET,[49] recommended by Kappesser who noted in a patient that the use of soft soap in the treatment of scabies caused glandular swellings in the neck to disappear. Since that time it has been advised and employed by many observers.

KÜLBS [50] states that this therapy has shown many brilliant results in the treatment of glandular tuberculosis. HOFFA [51] in 1899 noticed the increased appetite and general well-being as well as the resorption of the tuberculous glands incident to this form of treatment. In recent times Kousch has brought forth the soap treatment and claims it to be very good in treating tuberculosis. KÜLBS rubs a tablespoonful of green soap into the skin of the extremities and trunk every six days, changing the place of inunciation at each rubbing. He rubs for about five minutes, lets the skin dry for three to five minutes and then washes it off with lukewarm water. By so doing he does not see irritation of the skin or eczema following the treatment. Others employ a different technique, some applying the soap more often, every day or every other day. Some allow the soap to remain for a quarter to a half hour, others apply it at night, and do not wash it off until morning. More energetic methods are applicable in case of adults because of the harder skin.

Modes of Action not Known.—The exact mode of action of the soap treatment for tuberculous lesions is not clear. Green soap is a combination of potassium and various fatty acids. When applied to the skin it causes a softening of the epidermis and more vigorous application leads to erythema and irritation of the skin. The location of the tuberculous process does not seem to be of consequence in deciding the site of application of soap. The value of the treatment has been attested to by HAUSSMAN, KLINGELHOEFFER, SENATOR, KOLLMAN, CORNET and others.[52] This treatment is simple and easily employed anywhere and may be used even for the poorest, and if it is of any value it merits some consideration. This form of treatment would seem to be very inadequate in view of the now recognized nature of the enlargement and would not be considered, but for the reputation of the investigators reporting success in its use.

BIBLIOGRAPHY

CHAPTERS I, II and III

ANATOMY AND PHYSIOLOGY

1. F. R. Sabin: Am. Journal of Anatomy. 1904-'05, 4.
2. Delamere, Poirier and Cuneo: The Lymphatics.
3. A. Most: Die Topographi des Lymphgefàssapparates des Kopfes und des Halses. 1906.
4. P. Bartels: Das Lymphgefässystem. 1909.
5. Henkle: Arch. f. Laryngologie und Rhinologie. 1914, Bd. 28, Ht. 2, p. 231.
6. K. Amersbach: Arch. f. Laryngologie und Rhinologie. 1914, Bd. 29, Ht. 1, p. 29.
7. G. B Wood· Tonsillar Infection. Therap. Gazette. 1915, 3rd s. XXXI, p 83.
8. W. S. Miller: The Anatomical Record. Vol. 5, No. 3. The American Journal of Roentgenology, 1917, June.
9. W. S. Miller: Bulletin of the Robert Koch Society for the Study of Tuberculosis, 1913-1916.
10. R. Tigerstedt: Lehrbuch der Physiol. des Menschen, 1913.
11. Carlson, Grear and Becht: Amer. Journal of Phys. Boston, 1908, 22.
12. Carlson, Grear and Luckhard: *Ibid*.
13. Starling: Principles of Human Physiology, 1912.
14. Luciani: Human Physiology. 1911.

CHAPTER IV

ETIOLOGY

1. Bandelier and Roepke: A Clinical System of Tuberculosis. .
2. Much, H.: Die nach Ziehl nicht darstellbaren Formen d. Tb. Bz. Berlin, klin. Wochenschr. 1988, p. 691.

3. Quoted from Bandelier and Roepke: A Clinical System of Tuberculosis.
4. Quoted from Baldwin: Etiology of Tuberculosis. Osler and
   McCrae.
5. *Ibid.*
6. Quoted from McFarland: Text-book upon the Pathogenic Bacteria.
7. Quoted from Baldwin: Etiology of Tuberculosis. Osler and
   McCrae.
8. Chabas: Deux erreurs de la phthisiologie: La predisposition et
   l'hérédité Revue internat. de la tuberculose. 1914, Vol.
   XXV, p. 79.
9. Quoted from Baldwin: Etiology of Tuberculosis. Osler and
   McCrae.
10. Theobald Smith: Transactions, Assn. Amer. Phys. 1896, XI,
    p. 75.
11. G. Cornet: Scrofulosis, 2nd Ed.
12. Duval: Journal of Exper. Med. XI, 1909.
13. Quoting from Much, H.: Die Immunitäts-wissenschaft. 1914.
14. G. Cornet: Die Tuberculose, 2nd. Ed.
15. Park: Congr. of Hyg. and Demography. 1912, Wash. Vol. IV,
    267.
16. A. P. Mitchell: The Journal of State Med. 1915, XXIII, p. 1.
    Journal of Path. and Bact. 1917, XXI.
17. Woodhead: Tr. XV, Internat. Congr. Hyg. and Demography.
    1912, Wash. Vol. IV, 252
18. Copeland: VI. Int. Congr. on Tuberculosis. 1908, II, 379.
19. Quoting from Copeland: *Ibid.*
20. Young: Journal of State Med. 1915, XXIII, 21.
21. Quoting from G. Thompson: Medical Press and Circular. 1913,
    95, p. 33.
22. Baldwin: *Loc. cit.*
23. Quoted from Clopper: Arch. of Ped. 1915, XXXII, 843.
24. Manning and Knott: Am. Journal of Dis. Child. 1915, X, 354.
    Rosquist: Finska läkaresällskapets förhandl. 1913, LV (1), p.
    186.
25. Manning and Knott: *Loc. cit.*
26. Fishberg: Arch. of Ped. 1915, XXXII, p. 20.
27. Manning and Knott: *Loc. cit.*
28. H. Brown: A. Journal Abst. 1913, 68.

29. Wollstein and Bartlett: Am. Journal of Dis. of Child. 1914, 8, p. 362.

30. Quoted: *Ibid.*

31. Rothe: Deutsche med. Woch. 1911, XXXVII, I, 343.

32. J. L. Morse: Boston M. and S. Journal. 1915, CLXXIII, p. 655.

33. O. Medin: Arch. f. Kinderh. 1913, 61, p. 482.

34. Quoted from Rothe: *Loc. cit.*

35. Rothe: *Loc. cit.*

36. Wollstein and Bartlett: *Loc. cit.*

37. Hedren: Zeitschr. f. Hyg. und Infekt. 1913, 73, p. 273.

38. Quoted from A. Most: Die Topographic des Lymphgefässapp. des mensch. Korp. etc. Bibl. med. Abt. C, Heft, 21.

39. Cornet: Scrofulosis, 2nd Ed.

40. Quoted from K. Hochsinger: Kassowitz, Festschrift. 1912. G. Cornet: Scrofulosis. Engel: Med. Kl. Berlin. 1913, IX, 2099.

41. Quoted from O. Heubner: Lehrbuch der Kinderheilkunde. G. Cornet: Scrofulosis.

42. O. Heubner: Lehrbuch der Kinderheilkunde.

43. B. Salge: Scrofula, The Diseases of Children. Ed. by Pfaundler and Schlossman.

44. K. Hochsinger: Was ist Scrofulose? Kassowitz, Festschrift. 1912.

45. Quoted from B. Salge: *Loc. cit.*

46. E. Smith: Disease in Children.

47. Holt: Diseases in Infancy and Childhood.

48. Baldwin: Etiology of Tuberculosis. Osler and McCrae.

CHAPTER V

PATHOLOGY

1. Calmette: Revue de la tuberculose. 1913, No. 5, 321.

2. Quoting from Calmette: *Ibid.*

3. G. Cornet: Scrofulosis, 2nd Ed. 1914.

4. F. Harbitz: Münch. med. Woch. 1913, IX, p. 741.

5. Quoting from W. H. Park: Arch. of Ped. 1915, XXXII, 485.

6. G. Cornet: Scrofulosis, 2nd Ed. 1914.

7. Quoting from Baldwin: Et. of Tuberculosis. Osler and McCrae.

8. Medin: *Loc. cit.*
9. Quoting from Bandelier and Roepke: A Clinical System of Tuberculosis, 2nd Ed. 1913.
10. Zarfl: Jahrb. f. Kinderh. 1913, LXXVII, p. 95.
11. Quoted from Stoll and Heublein: Am. Journal of M. Sc. Phil. 1914, 148, p. 369.
12. C. Hedrén: *Loc. cit.*
13. A. Ghon: Der primäre Lungenherd bei der Tub. der Kinder. 1912.
14. Quoting from Calmette: *Loc. cit.*
15. Wollstein and Bartlett: *Loc. cit.*
16. Calmette: Revue de la tuberculose. 1913, No. 35, 321.
17. Quoting from Calmette: *ibid.*
18. L. Findley: Br. Journal Ch. Dis. 1913, X, 502.
19. Walsham: The Channels of Infection in Tuberculosis.
20. v. Pirquet: Edinb. M. Journal. 1914, 13, p. 220.
21. G. Cornet: Scrofulosis, 2nd Ed. 1914.
22. Cobbet: Br. Journal Ch. Dis. 1911, VIII, 415.
23. Quoting from Calmette: *Loc. cit.*
24. A. Ghon: *Loc. ctt.*
25. Quoting from G. Cornet: *Loc. cit.*
26. Hedrén: *Loc. cit.*
27. Quoted from Woodhead: Tr. XV, Intern. Cong. Hyg. & Demogr. Wash. 1912, IV, 252.
28. Rothe: Deutsche med. Woch. 1911, XXXVII, I, 343.
29. Wollstein and Bartlett: *Loc. cit.*
30. W. H. Park: Congr. Hyg. and Demogr. Wash. 1912, IV, 267.
31. Quoted from Cornet: *Loc. cit.*
32. Mitchell: The Journal of State Med. 1915, XXIII, p. 1.
33. Woodhead: *Loc. cit.*
34. Quoted from Cornet: *Loc. cit.*
35. Gardiner: Lancet. 1915, 189, p. 752.
36. Lockard: Tuberculosis of the Nose and Throat.
37. G. B. Wood: Penn. Med. Journal, June. 1912.
38. Quoted from G. Cornet: *Loc. cit.*
39. Pybus: Lancet. 1915, 188, 1009.
40. Street: Journal of Ophth. Otology and Laryngology. 1915, 21, 141.
41. Quoted from Bandelier: Beiträge z Klin. der Tub. 1906, Bd. 6.
42. Gardiner: *Loc. cit.*
43. Quoted from Pybus: Lancet. 1915, 188, 1009.

44. Quoted from G. Cornet: Scrofulosis, 2nd Ed. 1914.
45. J. Grober: Klin. Jahrbuch. 1905, XIV.
46. Quoted from Pybus: *Loc. cit.*
47. Pybus: *Ibid.*
48. Blumenfield: Zeitschr. f. Laryng. u. Rhinol., etc. Bd. I, Ht. 4. 1908.
49. Quoted from Simon: Beitr. z. Klin. d. Tub. 1911, XIX, 417.
50. *Ibid:*
51. Calmette: *Loc. cit.*
52. Lockard: Tuberculosis of the Nose and Throat.
53. Walsham: *Loc. cit.*
54. Jousset: Pédiat. prat. 1914, XII, 208.
55. Medin: *Loc. cit.*
56. Blair: Surg. Gyn. and Obst. 1914, XVIII, 470.
57. H. Starck: Münch. med. Woch. 1896, XLIII, 145.
58. Quoted from Moorehead: J. A. M. A. 1910, 55-495.
59. *Ibid:*
60. Quoted from G. Cornet: *Loc. cit.*
61. H. Starck: *Loc. cit.*
62. Enler: Therapeut. Monatshefte, Berlin. 1915, XXIX, Sept.
63. Cook: Dental Review. 1899, XIII, 97.
64. Moorehead: J. A. M. A. 1910, 55, 495.
65. A. Moeller: Münch. med. Wochensch. 1910, No. 2.
66. Wright: Bost. Med. and Surg. Journal. 1915, 172, p. 8.
67. G. Cornet: Scrofulosis, 2nd Ed. 1914.
    Calmette: *Loc. cit.*
68. Bandelier and Roepke: A Clinical System of Tuberculosis.
69. Fordyce and Carmichael: Lancet, London. 1914, I, 25-26.
70. Bandelier and Roepke: *Loc. cit.*
71. Scheltema: Jahrb. f. Kinderh. 1914, LXXX, 118.
72. Chancellor: Zeitsch. f. Kinderh. (orig.). 1914, X, p. 12.
73. Jousset: Pédiat. prat. 1914, XII, 208.
74. A. Most: *Loc. cit.*
75. E. Holt: J. A. M. A. 1913, 61, p. 99.
76. Durck and Hektoen: Handbook of General Pathology.
77. Bartel: Quoted by Cornet: Scrofulosis, 2nd. Ed.
78. Holt: Diseases of Infancy and Childhood.
79. A. J. Mitchell: Jour. of Path. and Bact. 1917, XXI.
80. Eustace Smith: Chronic Tuberculosis. Practical Treatise on Diseases of Children.

CHAPTER VI

Symptoms

1. Edwards: Tuberculous Adenitis, Textbook of Medicine.
2. Quoted by Cornet: Nothnagel's Encyclopedia of Practical Medicine, American Edition.
3. See Cunningham's Anatomy, 1913, p. 1012.
4. Northrup, Quoted by Edwards: Textbook of Medicine.
5. Wollstein: Archives of Internal Medicine, 1909, III, 221.
6. Schick: Weiner klin. Wchsch. 1910, XXIII, p. 153.
7. Stoll: Am. Journal Dis. Children 1912, IV, 342.
8. Warthin: Osler & McCrae, System of Medicine.
9. Eustace Smith: Practical Treatise on Diseases of Children.
10. Petruschky: Münch. med. Wchschr. 1903, I, 364.
11. Riviere: Brit. Med. Journal. 1914, No. 280, p. 462.
12. Bing: Ugesk f. laeger. 1910, LXXII, p. 199.
13. Phillipi ⎫
14. Nagel ⎬ Quoted by Stoll: Am. Jour. Dis. Child. 1912, IV,
15. Krämer ⎪ p. 333
16. Phillipi ⎭
17. Smith: Wasting Diseases of Children. London, 1899, p. 309.
18. Cornet: Scrofulosis, p. 241.
19. Stoll: Am. Jour. Dis. Child. 1912, IV, p. 333.
20. D'Espine: Bulletin de l'acad. de med. Paris. 1907, LVII, 67.
21. Frazier: Old Dominion Jour. Med. & Surg. 1915, XXII, p. 63.
22. Morse: Boston Med. & Surg. Journal, CLXXIII, 654.
23. Howell: Am. Jour. Diseases of Children. 1915, X, 90.
24. Fishberg: Pulmonary Tuberculosis, p. 387.
25. Stoll: Am. Jour. Diseases of Children. 1912, IV, 333.
26. Wohlgemuth, quoted by Cornet: Nothnagel's Encyclopedia Practical Medicine.
27. Treves, Quoted by Holt: Diseases of Infancy and Childhood, p. 841.
28. Holt, Quoted by Holt: Diseases of Infancy and Childhood, p. 844.
29. A. P. Mitchell: Journal of Path. and Bact. 1917, XXI.
30. Quoted by Cornet: Nothnagel's Encyclopedia of Practical Medicine, American Edition.
31. Holt: Pediatrics. 1913, XXV, p. 315.

32. Dowd: Annals of Surgery. 1903.
33. Osler: Principles and Practice of Medicine, p. 176.
34. Lexer: Text Book of Surgery, p. 411.

CHAPTER VII

PROGNOSIS

1. Hutinel: Le pronostic des adenopathies tub. du mediastin. chez
l'enfant Revue de la tuberculose, Paris. 1914, 2 S, XI.

CHAPTER VIII

DIAGNOSIS

1. Dunham and Wolman: Johns Hopkins Hospital, Bulletin. 1911,
XXII, p. 231.
2. Bandelier and Roepke: Clinical System of Tuberculosis.
3. Zieler, Wolff-Eisner, Bandler & Kribick, Pick, Daels, Arondale &
Falk, Quoted by Cornet: Scrofulosis, p. 253.
4. Veeder and Johnson: Amer. Jour. Diseases of Children. 1915,
IX, p. 481.
5. Pottenger: Tuberculin in Diagnosis and Treatment, p. 35.
6. Tice: Ill Med. Journal. 1909, N. S. 16, 291.
7. Bandelier and Roepke: Lehrb. d. spez. Diagn. und Ther. d. tub.
1915.
8. Lowenstein & Kaufman: Zeitschrift f. Tub. Bd. X, Heft. 1.
9. Pottenger: Tuberculin in Diagnosis & Treatment, p. 27.
10. Bandelier and Roepke: Lehrb. d. spez. Diagn. und Therap. d.
Tub. 1915.
11. Sahli: Tuberculin Treatment, pp. 145-6.
12. Sahli: Tuberculin Treatment, p. 85.
13. Besredka et Jupiele: Ann. de l'inst. Pasteur, Paris. 1913, XXVII,
1009.
Besredka et Manquknine: Compt. rend. de la soc. de biol. Paris.
1914, LXVI, 180-197.
14. McIntosh & Fildes: Lancet. 1914, II, 485.
15. Bronfenbrenner: Arch. int. med. XIV, p. 786.

16. Craig: Amer. Jour. Med. Sc. 1915, 150, II, p. 781.
17. Kinghorn & Twitchell: Amer. Jour. Med. Science. 1909, N. S. Vol. 137, p. 404.

CHAPTER IX

TREATMENT

1. A. F. Hess: J. A. M. A. 1914, LXIII, 2176.
2. M. E. Lapham: N. Y. Med. Journal. 1915, 101, p. 108.
3. Sahli's Tuberculin treatment. Dr. H. Sahli. 1912.
4. Tuberculin Therapy. F. M. Pottenger, Med. Recorder, Feb. 20, 1915.
5. Pottenger: *Ibid.*
6. Quoted from Bandelier and Roepke: A Clinical System of Tuberculosis.
7. Quoted from H. Much: Die Immunitatswissenschaft. 1914.
8. Bullock: Br. Journal of Tub. 1915, IX, 126.
9. Quoted from Kolmer: Infection, Immunity and Spec. Therapy.
10. Quoted from Sahli's Tuberculin Treatment.
11. Quoted from Bushnell: Military Surgeon. 1913, XXXII, 29.
12. Bullock: *Loc. cit.*
13. H. Much: Die Immunitätswissenschaft. 1914.
14. F. C. Smith: J. A. M. A. 1916, LXVI, 77.
15. Wasserman and Bruck: Quoted from Sahli's Tuberculin Treatment.
16. Sahli's Tuberculin Treatment, p. 131.
17. Cornet. Scrofulosis, p. 250.
18. Wolff-Eisner: Zentralblatt fr Bakteriologie, XXXVII, S. 3–455. Berl. klin. Woch. 1904, Nos. 42–44 (quoted by Sahli).
19.
20. Recent Advances in Knowledge of Allergic Phenomena. Ed-
21. itorial J. A. M. A. 1915, LXV, p. 2240.
22.
23. Bandelier and Roepke: Lehrbuch der spez. Diagn. u. Therap. der Tub. 1915.
24. Quoted from Bandelier and Roepke: Wilms, Deut. med. Wochenschr. 1911, No. 36.
25. Dautwis: Beiheft z. med. Klin. 1908, Ht. 9.

26. Hamman and Wollman: Tuberculin in Diagnosis and Treatment.
   Ager: Am. Journal Obst. 1911, LXIII, 368.
   Stoll: Am. Journal Med. Science. 1911, CXLI, 83.
   Philip: Lancet. 1909, II, 19.
   Griswold: Northwest Med. 1911, III, 189.
27. Pirie: Proceedings Royal Society Medicine. 1909-10, Vol. II,
   Part 1, Electrotherapeutic Section.
28. Broca & Mahar: Strahlentherapie. 1914, 4.
29. Kienboeck: Quoted by Skinner.
   Pirie: Interstate Med. Journal. 1914, XXI, 483.
30. Kienboeck: Roentgen-Taschenbuch. 1911, Bd. III, 96.
31. H. Mowat: British Med. Journal. 1914, II, p. 11.
32. O. H. Petersen: Strahlentherapie. 1914, IV, 272.
33. Tixier: Strahlentherapie. 1914, IV, 272.
34. Tonsey: Treatment of Tuberculous Glands of Neck. Medical
   Electricity & X-ray, p. 1080.
35. Iselin: Quoted by Petersen, Therapie der Gegenwart. 1914, LV,
   145.
36. Philipowiez: Wien. klin. Woch. 1913, XXVI, 2106.
37. Iselin: Deutsch, Zeitschr f. Chir. Vol. 103, p. 483.
38. Roques: Arch. d'electric med. Vol. 21, No. 333, p. 57.
39. O. H. Petersen: Die Therapie der Gegenwart. 1914, LV, 145.
40. Fritsch: Münch. med. Woch. 1913, LX, 2610.
41. Blaisch: Ergebn der Chir. und Orthop. 1913, VII, 111.
42. von Mutsenbacher: Quoted by Johnson's Therapeusis, Vol. III,
   385.
43. Bergonie: Compt. rend. Acad. des sciences, Paris. 1905, 140, 889.
44. Jesionek: Zeitschrift f. Tuberk. 1915, XXIV, No. 6.
45. O. H. Petersen: Therapie der Gegenwart. 1914, LV, 145.
46. Dietrich: Journal American Medical Assn. LXI, 2229.
47. Hirscb: American Journal Obstetrics. 1913, V. 68, p. 370.
48. G. B. Webb: Journal of Outdoor Life. 1915, XII, No. 9, 277.
49. Cornet: Scrofulosis, p. 385.
50. Kulbs: Therapeutische Monatshefte, 1914, 28, 661.
51. Hoffa, quoted by Kulbs: Ibid.
52. Haussman, Klingelhoeffer, Senator, Kollman: Quoted by Cornet:
   Scrofulosis, p. 386.

INDEX

Printed in the United States of America

Tuberculosis of the Bones and Joints in Children

By JOHN FRASER, M.D., F.R.C.S.E., Ch.M.,
Assistant Surgeon, Royal Hospital for Sick Children, Edinburgh

With 51 full page plates (2 in color) and 164 figures in the text.
Royal 8vo, 352 pp., index, $4.50

Tuberculous disease of the bones and joints is in large measure a disease of children, and as a result of the disastrous consequences which so often follow its course, it is one of the most important of the various forms of Tuberculosis. This work deals fully with the condition. The more recent investigations on the Etiology are fully discussed, the Pathology is a special feature, and much of the material in this relation is original. Diagnosis, Prognosis and Treatment are fully discussed. Special attention has been paid to the making and fitting of the various splints.

Dr. Fraser is well known to American physicians through his various magazine contributions and lectures. His book is without doubt one of the most important publications that has yet appeared on this subject.

THE MACMILLAN COMPANY
Publishers   64–66 Fifth Avenue   New York

Infection and Resistance

An Exposition of the Biological Phenomena underlying the Occurrence of Infection from Infectious Disease.

By HANS ZINSSER, M. D.

Major, Medical Officers' Reserve Corps, U. S. A.; Professor of Bacteriology at the College of Physicians and Surgeons, Columbia University, New York

With a Chapter on Colloids and Colloidal Reactions

By PROFESSOR STEWART W. YOUNG, Department of Chemistry, Stanford University

New Second Edition, completely revised.

Crown 8vo, ill., bibliography, index, 585 pp., $4.25

Since the publication of the first edition of this book, four years ago, it has been accepted as the standard work on the subject in our language and has been termed the "classic on Immunity in all languages."

The book has been rewritten and entirely reset and all important changes necessitated by the lapse of time have been made, also much new material has been added.

The chapters on *Anaphylaxis* have been almost completely rewritten. The Abderhalden reaction having been proved to be an interesting camouflage, the material in that section has been revised and the more recent work on *Enzymes* added. The development of conceptions of non-specific serum and cellular reactions has been discussed, while a section on *Immunity in Syphilis* has been added and the chapter dealing with specific therapy in various infections has been revised and expanded. In addition, many other alterations and comments have been made.

THE MACMILLAN COMPANY

Publishers   64–66 Fifth Avenue   New York

The Treatment of Acute Infectious Diseases

By FRANK SHERMAN MEARA, M.D.

Professor of Therapeutics, Cornell Medical School

Cloth, 8vo, $4.00

A widely known teacher has written this book along new and very unusual lines. The chapters deal with individual diseases in a thoroughly practical manner, each little detail of procedure being explained so that the reader may actually apply it. The reason for each procedure as based on our latest information is given with respect to both physical therapy and drugs.

Of especial importance is the *Summary at the end of each chapter*, where the most important points of the chapter are tabulated for the use of the student's review and for the busy practitioner. In this way procedures that necessarily must be referred to again and again will have separate consideration and will be referred to in the individual instances. All material is thus immediately at hand without constant reference to other sources or other parts of the book. The work is unique in its conception and the material is authoritative in every way.

THE MACMILLAN COMPANY

Publishers   64-66 Fifth Avenue   New York

Typhoid Fever

CONSIDERED AS A PROBLEM OF SCIENTIFIC MEDICINE

By FREDERICK P. GAY

Professor of Pathology in the University of California

Cloth, 8vo, $2.50

"In this book the author undertakes to deal with typhoid fever as a problem of scientific medicine rather than to handle it as a question solely of the clinic or of the laboratory. The point of view is broad and the treatment, on the whole, well balanced. The treatise illustrates one of the newer tendencies in American medicine, and, it is to be hoped, will prove a forerunner of other books on special topics which shall not only give critical surveys of the enormous mass of accumulated research, much of which may otherwise remain unassimilated and valueless, but shall also stimulate investigation by pointing out unsettled questions. . . .

"As might be anticipated from the author's own work, the chapters on immunization, the practical aspects of vaccination, and vaccine and serum treatments are particularly full and discriminating. The chapter on the carrier condition and the section dealing with laboratory diagnosis of typhoid are also informed throughout by the author's own personal experience. . . . The book has a good bibliography."—*Journal of American Medical Association.*

"The author has presented in this small volume an excellent exposition of the problem of typhoid fever. . . . It treats historically the development and present status of our knowledge concerning this important malady as viewed from the standpoint of its mechanism. . . . It shows the very close relationship between the clinical and the laboratory side of the disease by following the life history of the typhoid bacillus rather than the manifestations of the disease it produces. . . . The chapter on the protective value of vaccination against typhoid fever and the statistics relative to same are most interesting reading."—*New Orleans Medical & Surgical Journal.*

THE MACMILLAN COMPANY

Publishers   64–66 Fifth Avenue   New York

Milton Keynes UK
Ingram Content Group UK Ltd.
UKHW012013010224
437136UK00005B/162

9 781020 773211